# For The Beauty:

How Our Food Choices Affect God's World

Jennifer Moore MS, RD, CSR, NSCA-CPT

For the beauty of the earth,
For the beauty of the skies,
For the love which from our birth
Over and around us lies,
Lord of all, to thee we raise
This our grateful hymn of praise.

For the beauty of each hour
Of the day and of the night,
Hill and vale, and tree and flower,
Sun and moon and stars of light,
Lord of all, to thee we raise
This our grateful hymn of praise.

For the joy of human love,
Brother, sister, parent, child,
Friends on earth, and friends above,
Pleasures pure and undefiled,
Lord of all, to thee we raise
This our grateful hymn of praise.

For each perfect gift of Thine,
To our race so freely given,
Graces human and divine,
Flowers of earth and buds of heaven,
Lord of all, to thee we raise
This our grateful hymn of praise.

For thy Church which evermore
Lifteth holy hands above,
Offering up on every shore
Her pure sacrifice of love,
Lord of all, to thee we raise
This our grateful hymn of praise.

# Contents

# Acknowledgements

Much Love and Thanks To:

My amazing husband Chad Moore who supports me in every endeavor, including this book. Chad, a Master Sergeant in our United States Air Force, displays strength and leadership in all he does. That being said, he has shown me that a strong man is also one who cherishes his wife. He embraced plant based nutrition displaying that strength is teachable and willing to look at the facts. Thank you for being the man I never dreamed existed.

My babies, Sam, Hannah, Nate, and soon to be baby Steven. You inspire me to be more. You bring joy into my life with every thought of you.

My Lord and Savior Jesus Christ. I am nothing apart from You. You are my righteousness, strength, honor, wisdom, joy, peace, life. Thank You for saving my soul, sanctifying my life, and using me to better Your kingdom. I do not deserve Your mercy.

# Introduction

"The thief comes to steal, kill and destroy, but I have come
that they may have life and have it to the full."
—John 10:10

"Just read the book." This is the closing remark my teacher
gave at a vegetarian nutrition class when I interned at
Vanderbilt University Medical Center. She stated this after
our program's director gave her a disapproving glance.
Why might the director dislike her direction with the
course? Because she had been discussing material covered
from an unconventional book. Themes revealed ethical
issues surrounding meat consumption, a controversial
topic for that era. The book she referenced was *Diet for a
New America* by John Robbins. Her class intrigued me.
Being from Mississippi, I had never thought about
excluding meat from my diet—until then. I wanted the
truth, so I read the book. Then I became a vegetarian.

Once I had completed the internship and become a
registered dietitian, I moved back to Mississippi. My
newfound lifestyle met with disapproval in my southern
surroundings, to say the least. Most people considered me
weird, fanatic, and overboard. Feeling like an outsider, I
asked myself, why was I being criticized for something that
improved my health? Needless to say, I remained
vegetarian for a time, and then I phased in and out of
eating meat.

After the birth of my third child, I faced the fact that my
food choices and values did not align. I knew it was time to
return to a plant-based diet. I began to think more about
what I would feed my children and teach them about
food. I knew I did not want them to think of the typical

Western diet as being good. I wanted them to know the truth, and this desire grew even stronger as they aged.

The truth is, the typical American diet loaded with animal protein and fat has consequences. It creates three tragedies: an act of cruelty toward God's creatures, destruction of God's environment, and a degradation of his people's health. Allow me to teach you how typical American eating habits contribute to these three calamities. Let me share with you the truth that vegetarian nutrition positively impacts God's world: his creatures, the environment, and his people's health. What you do with the truth is your decision, but it's important that you get the information.

German philosopher Arthur Schopenhauer once said, "All truth goes through three stages; first it is ridiculed. Then it is violently opposed. Finally it is accepted as self-evident." I believe that God's people should consider their diet when reflecting on a relationship with him. If you really think about what you read in this book, I imagine you will change the way you eat. I pray that you will look with an open mind at the evidence provided in this book. I pray you develop a love for animals beyond the ones that may live in your home. I pray you slow down and look at God's world with awe and wonder. I pray you begin to desire to protect these gifts and the gift of your own health while you live your life to the fullest.

# Disclaimer

My goal is not to make new rules for people to follow so they be like the Pharisees and act superior. I don't hope to end up encouraging self-righteous Pharisees to make meat eaters feel like unrighteous sinners. No, that is not my vision. I simply ask Christians to become more aware of the meat and dairy industry's practices. Readers can then decide how and what to feed themselves and their families. Take a look at Romans 14 for a few minutes and then 1 Corinthians 10:23-24. Note how Romans speaks against judging others.

**Romans 14**

"Accept the one whose faith is weak, without quarreling over disputable matters. One person's faith allows them to eat anything, but another, whose faith is weak, eats only vegetables. The one who eats everything must not treat with contempt the one who does not, and the one who does not eat everything must not judge the one who does, for God has accepted them. Who are you to judge someone else's servant?"

My goal is education, not judgment. The following pages provide evidence that goes beyond religious convictions over whether to choose meat versus vegetables. Think about your diet. If you eat meat ask yourself: where did it come from? How was it raised? Were the animals treated in a way in which Jesus would approve? If not, how do you feel about contributing to bad practice? What is eating meat doing to your health? How is it affecting the environment? Ask God for direction. Then make a decision how to proceed with your life.

## Giving an Account on Big Issues-Romans Continued

"So then, each of us will give an account of ourselves to God."

"I am convinced, being fully persuaded in the Lord Jesus, that nothing is unclean in itself. But if anyone regards something as unclean, then for that person it is unclean."

"For the kingdom of God is not a matter of eating and drinking, but of righteousness, peace and joy in the Holy Spirit, because anyone who serves Christ in this way is pleasing to God and receives human approval."

I am not referring to "unclean" in the context of these verses. You will see through the atrocities revealed in this book that factory farming destroys God's earth. It also devastates His people. Righteousness, peace, and joy cannot coincide with the meat industry's practices.

"Let us therefore make every effort to do what leads to peace and to mutual edification. Do not destroy the work of God for the sake of food."

"So whatever you believe about these things keep between yourself and God. Blessed is the one who does not condemn himself by what he approves. But whoever has doubts is condemned if they eat, because their eating is not from faith, and everything that does not come from faith is sin."

As you read through the pages of this book, I pray you will examine what you believe and what you practice in light of the knowledge you gain.

1 Corinthians 10:23-24

A transition to 1 Corinthians 10:23-24 seals the foundation of my vision. These verses are presented in several versions:

New International Version: "I have the right to do anything, you say-but not everything is beneficial. "I have the right to anything"-but not everything is constructive. No one should seek their own good, but the good of others.

Easy to Read Version: "All things are allowed,' you say. But not all things are good. 'All things are allowed.' But some things don't help anyone. Try to do what is good for others, not just what is good for yourselves."

Bible in Basic English: "We are free to do all things, but there are some things which it is not wise to do. We are free to all things, but not all things are for the common good."

Eating animal products is not inherently sinful behavior. However a meat-and-dairy centered diet does not benefit the common good. Research verifies this. I cannot keep to myself the awareness that I have attained over the years; that is not an option. We live in community. I must seek the good of all. Choosing a plant-based diet is a relevant issue for God's people today.

God, I pray that you use me to help others.

# Chapter 1

## Blinding Distress

Concern for animals is a matter of taking the side of the weak against the strong, something the best people have always done.

—Harriet Beecher Stowe

**Blinded So He Could See.**

The older we become, the more we get set in our ways. We assume the way we were raised was based on truth. If that truth is now challenged, it may require us to change, so we turn a blind eye rather than face the change we might have to make.

This concept characterizes human nature. Remember the Israelites? They looked back to Egypt: "For it would have been better for us to serve the Egyptians than that we should die in the wilderness." They feared change—the unknown—so much so that they desired slavery. They could not open their eyes to the truth that God was leading and loving them.

The apostle Paul epitomized adherence to the way he had been reared. In his own words, "Men and brethren, I am a Pharisee, the son of a Pharisee" (Acts 23:6). Raised a Pharisee, he killed for what he believed. In the words of others prior to his transformation, "As for Saul, he made havoc of the church, entering every house, and dragging off men and women, committing them to prison" (Acts 8:3). Jesus changed Paul on the road to Damascus when Jesus spoke to him and blinded him. Paul converted to Christianity when he was shown the truth by Ananias: "There fell from his eyes something like scales, and he received sight at once; and he arose and was baptized" (Acts 9:18). He completely transformed after his eyes were opened, and he was no longer blind. Paul began worshiping Jesus; this is remarkable since he was trying to wipe out the believers in Jesus just three days before his conversion.

As Christians, we need to put ourselves in the situation of Paul. We need to consider the truth of animal agriculture to decide if change is necessary. We cannot accomplish this if we are blind, so prepare to  let the scales fall.

## Certainty

Why do you eat the way you do? Do you really know what you are eating, or do you just eat it because you always have eaten this way? We all have images surrounding food that bring comfort. Think about the terms "farm," "milk," "cookies," "home-cooked meal," "grilled-cheese sandwich," "chicken noodle soup," "biscuits," and "fried chicken." The foods seem peaceful. Now let's take another look at these words.

## Farming Today

The word "farm" typically conjures up images of open grassy fields with cattle grazing, a red barn with a weather vane on top, and chickens pecking the ground. You know the image. Now let's step into 2012. Today's farm could be better described as a large industrial facility, a factory, or a manufacturing plant. Our government refers to these so-called farms as Concentrated (or Confined) Animal Feeding Operations (CAFO).[1] These CAFOs degrade God's creatures, which directly defies God's command to humans regarding animals.

## They Are Mine

Genesis 1:26 gives people charge over animals: "Then God said 'Let Us make man in Our image, according to Our likeness; let them have dominion over the fish of the sea, over the birds of the air, and to everything that creeps on the earth in which there is life." What did God intend when he gave people dominion over the animals? Did the animals become ours, or do they still belong to God? The truth is, they are not ours. The word "dominion" refers to governance, not ownership. It's God who is the owner: "All the animals in the forest are mine and the cattle on thousands of hills. All the wild birds are mine and all living things in the field,"(Ps 50:10, 11).

We are stewards of God's creatures the same way we are with money, time, our children, and everything else on this earth. We do not own any of them. God created every animal and "was pleased" with what he had done (Gn 1:25). If good friends asked you to watch their dog while they went on vacation, how careful would you be with that dog? Now let me ask: how do we treat God's animals that he placed in our care—all of them? We might be nice to our pets, but on the other hand, how does our diet contribute to animal abuse?

## Let the Scales Fall

Proverbs 12:10 "The righteous care for the needs of their animals, but the kindest acts of the wicked are cruel"

Followers of Christ are vehemently against cruelty. Most, however, are unaware of the cruelty behind a meat-based diet.

The following images may disturb you. Much like Paul in his conversion and ultimate realization of the effect of his actions, turning a blind eye to reality is not an option. You see, God loves his animals. Luke 12:6 makes this clear when he writes of sparrows that "not one of them is forgotten before God." God fashioned each one with special characteristics, mannerisms, and habits. Please let the scales fall from your eyes as you read the next few pages about God's beautiful creatures. Appeal to your heart and your humanity.

## Pigs

Pigs are such amazing creations of God. After studying their God-given nature, I have come to regard them as one of my favorite animals. Read, and then discover the reality of pigs as I did.

Ken Kephart, a Penn State professor of animal science, has worked with pigs for over twenty years. He states that "pigs are clever without a doubt." According to Kephart, pigs are known to work in pairs to open latches and escape their pens. They have also been known to open up the other pens to let their pig pals out. Other research has shown that pigs' lives are as socially complex as those of primates. They have excelled at playing video games that have proven difficult for young children. Mother pigs can be found singing to their piglets while nursing.[2, 3]

God designed pigs to be outdoors. They naturally graze, root, and intermingle with other pigs.[4]

W. H. Hudson states this about pigs:

> I have a friendly feeling towards pigs generally and consider them the most intelligent of beasts...I also like his attitude toward other creatures, especially man. He is not suspicious, or shrinkingly submissive, like horses, cattle, and sheep; not an impudent devil-may-care like the goat; nor hostile like the goose; nor condescending like the cat; nor a flattering parasite like the dog. He views us from a totally different, a sort of democratic standpoint as fellow citizens and brothers, and takes it for granted, or grunted, that we understand his language, and without servility or insolence He has a natural, pleasant, camerados-all or hail-fellow-well-met air with us.[5]

Farmers today do not share Hudson's or God's view of pigs.

## American Pigs—The Real World

In factory farms where pigs are raised for food—the pigs eaten by Americans—they are in total confinement where they never see the sun. Their prison constricts them so tightly they cannot even turn around. No bedding or hay is provided for their God-given practice of rooting. When crowded like this, the pigs become violent. They begin cannibalistic behaviors where they will bite each other's tails and rumps. These are the same animals we just discussed that would open gates to let each other free. The factory farmer's solution to this inconvenience is to cut off their tails and chip off part of their teeth with no anesthesia, a practice that is outlawed in Britain. Data from 2001 reveals that ninety-five million US pigs were raised for meat, and sixty-five million of those were raised on these factory farms.[6]

Pig farmers today have certainly lost sight of God's view of his creation. Even as far back as 1976, in an issue of the journal, *Hog Farm Management,* farmers were advised to "forget the pig is an animal. Treat him just like a machine in a factory."[6] This statement should repulse Christians and stir up anger in our souls. God did not create the pig to be a machine.

Consider a more recent incident documented from the Humane Farming Association in the 2001 book, *The Food Revolution* by John Robbins:

> PETA recently obtained an undercover videotape of a North Carolina hog factory. The videotape depicts sows being beaten into and out of their crates with metal rods, disabled cows being kicked, stomped on, and dragged, sows killed by blows to the head with wrenches or cinderblocks, sows having their throats cut while fully conscious, and sows being skinned alive and having their legs

removed while still alive and moaning...Because "product uniformity" takes precedence over all else, thousands of pigs that don't make weight are killed. These animals are picked up by the hind legs and bashed head first into the concrete floor. Some companies call the process "thumping." Smithfield Farms (the nation's largest hog producer) calls it PACing—the company's acronym for "Pound Against Concrete"...The dead pigs are delivered to rendering plants where they are ground up and fed back to live pigs, cattle, and other animals.[7]

The dreadfulness continues with cows. Discover the reality of cows as I have.

**Cows**

God owns the "cattle on a thousand hills." God loves his creation. Cows are very relational animals, forming tight bonds with loved ones. Investigators report that cows become discernibly distressed when separated from those they love. This includes not only their cow families, but human companions as well.

Female cows are exceptionally maternal. If mother cows are separated from their young, as is common practice on factory farms, they stand and wait for their calves, even in harsh conditions. They have broken out of confinement and traveled miles to reunite with their young.[8]

Musician Kate Bush portrays it well: "People's general awareness is getting much better, even down to buying a pint of milk: the fact that the calves are actually killed so that the milk doesn't go to them but to us cannot really be right, and if you have seen a cow in a state of extreme distress because it cannot understand why its calf isn't by, it can make you think a lot."

Cows are maternal, loving, and unique. Did you know that God made each spot on a cow so unique that no two are alike?[8]

God took great care in his creation of this gentle beast.

**Great Care Denied**

Unfortunately, great care is not taken when humans raise cattle for food. Calves are taken from their mothers mere days after birth with the mother cows screaming for their young. How could Americans have milk, cheese, yogurt, and ice cream if the calf drank the mother cow's milk— which is God's design, by the way. You see, modern farms don't care about God's design. Remember, the farm is a factory and cows are just tools. In 1999, the *New York Times* ran an article on California dairy farms. One farm owner said she "never milked a cow by hand, and never expected to." She had Latinos and machinery for that job. She stated that "it's just a factory is what it is. If the cows don't produce milk, they go to beef."[9]

Cows are artificially impregnated yearly. Like humans, they too have nine-month gestation periods making them pregnant most of their short life. Though God created them to live up to twenty-five years, they are worthless to farmers beyond three to four years. By that time, they have been exhausted with multiple pregnancies and unnaturally large amounts of milk production due to injections with bovine growth hormone (BHG). They go to slaughter.

If God designed cow milk to be for calves then...?

## Baby Cows

So what happens to the calves that are torn away from their mothers? If the baby is male, he becomes veal. The veal process involves placing the calf in a small wooden box with a rope tied to his neck to restrict movement. He is deprived of sunlight and iron so that his meat will be pale and tender—abuse to produce a delicacy for the wealthy. Female calves follow the grueling path of their mothers.

So you are thinking, I cut red meat a long time ago. I am aware it is not good for my health. Sigh.

It is not time to relax yet. Let's move on to chickens.

### "I Eat Only Chicken—No Red Meat"

The above statement and practice that I encounter daily as a dietitian has led to a boom in the poultry industry. People believe erroneously that choosing chicken over beef is choosing the superior alternative. Facts reveal that chickens are regarded no higher than any other farm animal.

It is different with our Lord. Chickens are God's well thought-out creation.

The notion of chickens scratching and rooting for earthworms and grubs by the big red barn is an image from the past. Roosters are not crowing to wake up farmers and their families these days. Go on and imagine not a farm, but again a factory. Chickens are not seen as the handiwork of God. They have an imaginary dollar sign imprinted on their abused bodies.

CAFOs inflict chickens with pain just after birth. Each bird goes through a terrifying process known as debeaking. Don't worry. The Code of Practice only allows half of the upper beak and one third of the lower beak to be seared off by a hot blade.[11] Do we think that God would approve of this mutilation of his creatures? Do we think these creatures don't understand? The answer to both questions is a resounding no!

The hens do feel pain and understand fear, as they have to be captured and restrained by the farmer where their beaks are placed in the machine with the hot blade. The beaks of hens have cutaneous afferent nerves, so acute pain ensues. Additionally, the pain becomes chronic as the nerve fibers regenerate and tumors form. These tumors are known as "neuromas" and mimic the phantom limb pain experienced by humans who have had amputations.[10]

## Why Debeak?

The appalling conditions in which chickens are forced to live result in aggravated birds. Chickens have a God-given instinct towards a pecking order. Egg-producing hens are crammed into cages with so many other hens they cannot even spread their wings. Their tight confines cause them to become agitated and aggressive. They are not allowed to be what God created them to be. Of course they are frustrated! Thus farmers debeak them so that their aggression does no damage to their precious meat.[7]

## What about Chicks?

Male chicks are rubbish to factory farmers since they cannot lay eggs. They are put on an assembly line with their sisters where they are weeded out. From there, they are either thrown into a garbage bag to suffocate or thrown alive into a meat grinder and fed back to their mothers and sisters or other livestock. So, farmers sear off the beaks of chickens to prevent aggression and "cannibalism" then grind up their young to feed back to them? Isn't that...cannibalism? [7]

18

## Out of Confinement—On to Slaughter

Would you kill your pet dog or cat to eat it? How about an animal you're not emotionally attached to? Is the thought of slaughtering a cow or chicken or pig with your own hands too much to handle? Instead, would hiring a hit man to do the job give you enough distance from the emotional discomfort? What animal did you put a contract out on for your supper last night? Did you at least make sure that none went to waste and to take a moment to be grateful for its sacrifice? (Anonymous)

After living their God-given life in the wretched conditions, animals are slaughtered. It would be a slight consolation if this process were humane and quick, putting them out of their misery. It is not.

Open your eyes as we go behind the walls of American slaughterhouses.

## Glass Walls

Paul McCartney said wisely, "If a slaughterhouse had glass walls, everyone would be a vegetarian." America's slaughterhouses are anything but humane.

On March 4, 2009, Wayne Pacelle, President and CEO of The Humane Society of the United States testified to the House Oversight and Government Reform Committee, providing a view of what truly goes on behind the walls of slaughterhouses. He describes undercover footage of an investigation at the Hallmark/Westland Meat Packing Company in Chino, California. "Footage showed workers ramming cows with the blades of a forklift, jabbing them in the eyes, applying painful electric shocks often in sensitive areas, dragging them with chains pulled by heavy machinery, and torturing them with a high-pressure water hose to simulate drowning as they attempted to force these animals to walk to slaughter." At the time of this investigation, this very plant was second in provisions of beef to the National School Lunch Program. It had received honors in 2004–2005 by the USDA as "supplier of the year." This investigation resulted in the largest beef recall in history at Hallmark.[11] The USDA did shut the plant down as a result of the findings. However, how can a company that is supposedly regulated by our government be this inhumane? Unfortunately, this is not an uncommon occurrence.

According to federal law, mammals are to be stunned before being slaughtered to eliminate suffering. Frequent failed stuns are commonplace. Therefore, many animals do not have their neck cut before they regain consciousness while hanging from their legs on a bleed rail.[12]

One incident of a USDA inspector, supposedly the animal's advocate, laughed at a joke of a co-owner of slaughterhouse. An infant calf being sent to slaughter for "bob veal" staggered and fell into a trailer while covered in diarrhea. The co-owner jested that it looked like the USDA inspector on a Friday night; this is no laughing matter. Another USDA inspector was caught on tape watching as a worker skinned a calf alive.[11]

The accounts of abuse described are not the isolated instances that the animal agriculture business wants us to believe. I have read more reports that would take pages to describe to you. I am not the first to write about these cases of abuse. Many have gone before me as leaders and educators for animal welfare. In her book, *Slaughterhouse,* Gail A. Eisnitz presents many accounts of abuse. John Robbins describes similar examples in his books. PETA has conducted numerous undercover inspections revealing horrendous cruelty. Again, in the words of Wayne Pacelle, "Every time we have done an investigation at a slaughter plant or a livestock auction, we've found horrendous mistreatment."

So isn't there an agency overseeing slaughterhouses? Why yes there is.

## Mission Statements?

The Food Safety and Inspection Service (FSIS) is the Agency within USDA responsible for ensuring compliance with the Humane Methods of Slaughter Act. This Agency employs veterinarians and inspectors, but as we have seen in previous examples, many times these inspections fall short, to say the least. "The Food Safety and Inspection Service (FSIS) is the public health agency in the U.S. Department of Agriculture responsible for ensuring that the nation's commercial supply of meat, poultry, and egg products is safe, wholesome, and correctly labeled and packaged."[13] As you can see, the mission statement says absolutely nothing about animal welfare. The word "humane" is nowhere in the statement.

So if the government fails to follow through on its commitment to ensure that animals are treated humanely, what do we do? Do we stand for God's creation? Did he not place us in dominion over it? Let me ask again what it means to have dominion over the animals. What would it look like to be Christ-like regarding this issue? Let's look at God's character for that answer.

For starters, God cares for his animals.

## In His Hands

"You care for people and animals alike, O Lord" (Ps 36:6).

God feeds his animals, as you read in Matthew and the some of the psalms: "Look at the birds of the air, for they neither sow nor reap nor gather into barns, yet your heavenly Father feeds them" (Mt 6:26). "He gives the beast its food, and to the young ravens that cry" (Ps 147:9).

He has pity on his animals: "And should I not have concern for the great city of Nineveh, in which there are more than a hundred and twenty thousand people who cannot tell their right hand from their left—and also many animals?" (Jon 4:11). If God has pity on animals then could we not conclude that it is "Godly" to care for animals as well?

**He Expects His People to Do the Same**

We read again in Proverbs that "the Godly care for their animals, but the wicked are always cruel" (Prv 12:10).

God does not approve of animal abuse. Godly people should feel the same. Think for a minute about how most people respond with horror when they hear of animal abuse. Let me jog you memory about one incident. Remember the Michael Vick case? The NFL star was caught raising and violently abusing dogs for the "sport" of dog fighting. It was horrifying, and people were outraged. The media covered the story extensively and animal-rights groups jumped to action. Was this cruelty recognized only because the case involved dogs? The story was as distressing as the treatment of animals on factory farms and in slaughterhouses.

These animals do not live in our homes, so the media doesn't bother and people are less informed. However one day all animals will be protected in God's reign. God describes a peaceable kingdom in Isaiah 11:6 where "the wolf shall dwell with the lamb, and the leopard shall lie down with the kid; and the calf and the young lion and the fatling together; and a little child shall lead them." Again in the same chapter verse 2, you read that "the wolf and the lamb shall feed together, and the lion shall eat straw like the bullock; and dust shall be the serpent's meat. They shall not hurt nor destroy in all my holy mountain, saith the Lord."

These verses refer to the kingdom after Jesus returns to reign as king of kings. Do we not pray, "Thy kingdom come. Thy will be done on earth as it is in heaven"?

My prayer is that in every way possible I do not contribute to unnecessary pain and cruelty. As it will be in heaven, I want to be a part of a world where not only are people not abused, but also animals aren't abused.

God shows he cares for both. Again, Jonah 4:11 states, "And should I not have concern for the great city of Nineveh, in which there are more than a hundred and twenty thousand people who cannot tell their right hand from their left—and also many animals?"

God is the same yesterday, today, and forever. He cared for people and animals in the time of Jonah, and he still does today.

It is Godly to care for animals. It is right to be outraged at the treatment of farm animals. Pray for God's peaceable kingdom, and do your part to bring that kingdom to earth, as it is in heaven.

**Take-Home Messages and Tips**

**Change Your Habits**

How about changing the habits of your family to cut meat out of your diet partially or completely? Why do we have to serve hamburgers and hotdogs at every church function? Is that really okay? Could we try veggie dogs and burgers?

**Cast Your Vote**

Every time you purchase food, you are casting a vote. We live in a culture where demand dictates supply. If more people buy cheap meats and fast-food, these items will remain just that—cheap. If more people would buy fresh fruits, vegetables, dried beans and peas, and whole grains, these items will come down in price. The difference will be that they will still be quality, nutritious items—not cheap ones. Don't vote for the meat industry. Just simply stop promoting its cause. Why would we promote food that unmistakably demeans God's creatures?

**Teach Your Children Well...to Be Well**

More importantly, why do we feed our children this way? Adults feed children. Why would we teach them to eat this way? There are plenty of kid-friendly vegetables available now. See appendix D.

The above-mentioned ideas are options for sure, but we as Christians have a much more formidable weapon in our hands.

**Our Greatest Weapon**

How about prayer? What a simple measure we all can do. How about adding the humane treatment of animals to your prayer list along with other large-scale concerns? We pray for our country, wars, hunger, poverty, lawlessness, and the list goes on. Do you believe humane treatment of animals is important to God? Is it too edgy for Christian conservatives to care about? I think not. Don't we long for God's kingdom and pray to that end?

# Chapter 2

## Parched Land and Perishing Animals

How long will the land mourn, and the herbs of every
field wither? The beasts and birds are consumed,
 For the wickedness of those who dwell there.
—Jeremiah 12:4

## God's Environment

I remember a church I attended in Memphis, Tennessee made me very proud one Sunday in 2008. I was discussing with a friend the need to recycle church bulletins and how we as Christian should be the best environmentalists on the planet. The friend met my comment with scoff and ridicule. However, the very next Sunday the church announced the need to recycle, in order for us to be, as I said, the best environmentalists on the planet. I beamed with joy. That was a step in the right direction for sure, but what about the most potent polluter of air and water in the world. Do you know to what I am referring?

## More on Meat and Dairy

Take a look at these statistics:

- Amount of fossil fuels needed to produce a meat-centered diet versus a meat-free diet: three times more

- Number of acres of US forest cleared for cropland to produce a meat-centered diet: 260 million

- Amount of meat imported to the US annually from Central and South America: three hundred million pounds

- Area of tropical rainforest consumed in every quarter pound of rainforest beef: fifty-five square feet

- Current rate of species extinction due to destruction of tropical rainforest for meat grazing and other uses: one thousand per year

(http://www.consumercide.com/js/index.php/food-supply/39-necessarily-vegetarian.)

Were you aware of the impact of a meat centered diet? Are you concerned about the rainforests? I firmly believe we should be.

## Gifts to Treat with Care

The air we breathe, the water we drink, the temperature of our earth, animals, plants...each of these gifts wrought by God is easy to take for granted. They are so much a part of daily life that we can forget how precious they are. It may be hard to believe, but what we choose to eat can determine the size of the footprint we leave on this earth. Some of these footprints will cause great hardships for our children if we don't step lighter. Transforming our diet lessens our contribution to global warming and land and water devastation more than any other change we can make.

## Understanding Global Warming—Let's Begin Here

As a dietitian, I needed to research to understand the dynamic of global warming. I knew that our earth as we know it is changing due to global warming. I was also aware that the meat industry makes large contributions to our increased temperatures. Here is what I found.

## Greenhouse Gases

A greenhouse gas traps heat reflected from the earth in the atmosphere, preventing its escape into space. These gases benefit us in that they help warm our planet. The three main greenhouse gases to consider are carbon dioxide ($CO_2$), nitrous oxide ($N_2O$), and methane ($CH_4$).[1, 2] Each of these gases has what scientists refer to as "global warming potential" (GWP).

## Global Warming Potential

Global warming potential (GWP) refers to how much heat a greenhouse gas is capable of trapping in the atmosphere. Every environmental gas compares to carbon dioxide ($CO_2$) to calculate its relative GWP. $CO_2$, with a GWP of 1, is the most prevalent GHG, but the least powerful.[3]

## The Problem with Greenhouse Gases

The greenhouse effect is the retention of a portion of solar energy in the earth's atmosphere in the form of heat as a result of the presence of greenhouse gases.[4] As stated, God designed this beneficial warming mechanism. Without it, our earth would be 60 degrees Fahrenheit (F) colder, and we would all die. However, the amount of greenhouse gas in the atmosphere is too great mainly due to human activity or anthropogenic activity. Now we are experiencing a global climate change in the other direction.[2] It is too hot, and we should be concerned.

## Rising Temperatures—Who Cares?

The Environmental Protection Agency noted in 2009 that the ten warmest years recorded since 1850 have all occurred in the previous thirteen years. So besides just being plain hot, why should we care? That question may not be answered definitively. One speculation made by the Intergovernmental Panel on Climate Change (IPCC) states that by the year 2100 our earth will be 4.7 degrees Fahrenheit hotter.[5] Examples of consequences to our earth as it heats up are described by authors Gary Braasch and Bill McKibben:

"As a witness to climate change, I have stood in the empty rookeries of displaced Adelie penguins and felt the chill as huge icebergs separated from an ice shelf in Antarctica. I have seen jagged fronts of receding Greenland glaciers and observed subtle changes on the tundra. I have tracked down alpine glaciers depicted in 150-year-old images and rephotographed them to show them wasting away. In the woods of eastern North America I have walked among spring wildflowers and watched for migrant songbirds, which are arriving earlier each season than in decades past. Along the coast I have seen rising tides and heavy storms erode beaches. I have heard the anguish of voices of native Alaskans as they describe their village being washed away, of Chinese farmers facing famine caused by drought, and Pacific Islanders driven from their homes by increasingly high tides. Global warming is affecting the whole world from the tiniest plankton to humans in their cities and the flora and fauna of entire river basins and mountain ranges."[6]

## What's Meat Got to Do with It?

There are three main gases to consider when investigating GWP and global climate change. In addition to GWP, we must examine how long each gas remains in the atmosphere. This is depicted in "atmospheric lifetime" in table 1.  The longer a gas remains in the atmosphere, the greater the damage. Table 1 shows how much each of these gases contributes to the problem.

## TABLE 1: Power of Greenhouse Gases

| Gas | Carbon Dioxide Equivalent | Atmospheric Lifetime (years) |
|-----|---------------------------|------------------------------|
| Carbon dioxide ($CO_2$) | 1 | 50–200 |
| Methane ($CH_4$) | 21 | 10 |
| Nitrous oxide ($N_2O$) | 310 | 150 |

(As the table indicates, $CH_4$ is twenty-one times more effective at trapping heat in the atmosphere than $CO_2$.)

Regularly consumed animal products, e.g., beef, poultry, pork, dairy, and farmed seafood, contribute to global warming more than any other food product we consume. In fact, scientists estimate that animal agriculture accounts for approximately 60 percent of nitrous oxide emissions and approximately 50% percent of methane emissions.[7, 8, 9] Why is this?

Livestock contributes to GHG emissions both directly and indirectly.

**Gas-A Direct Method**

Livestock, particularly during cow digestion produces a natural by-product of methane gas. Yes—I am referring to belching and flatulence. You may be thinking: how can a cow with gas possibly be a significant contributor to global warming? A single cow would not be a significant contributor. The problem arises when greater than one billion ruminants reared annually have gas.[10]

**Direct Manure**

While we are on the subject of body processes, manure also raises concern. In the United States, around five hundred million tons of solid and liquid wastes are produced annually. Animal manure emits all three GHGs into the atmosphere.[11] In fact, 25 percent of agricultural methane emissions and 6 percent of nitrous oxide emissions can be credited to animal manure management.[12]

## Indirect Contributions—Feeding

Much of the world's crop production does not feed humans directly. It feeds animals that humans feed on later. The crops used to sustain livestock contribute to GHGs in several ways. First, crops must be fertilized. In the US, natural gas is the fuel used to produce nitrogen fertilizers from synthetically produced ammonia. The fertilizer must be packaged, transported, and applied. Natural gas and transportation contribute to $CO_2$ emissions. This initial phase of animal rearing accounts for 41 million tons of $CO_2$ emissions annually.[13]

Raising animals destroys our atmosphere. What about the earth where we reside?

## Land and Water

"And God called the dry land earth and the gathering of the waters He called seas. And God saw that it was good" (Gn 1:10). God gave humans a beautiful place to reside while we are mortal. Sadly, both the land and the water are spoiled largely due to animal agriculture.

## The Land God Gave Us—Deforestation

Deforestation creates more land to grow feed for animals or to house the animals themselves. The Food and Agriculture Organization of the United Nations reported in 2006 that raising livestock accounts for the use of 70 percent of all agricultural land and 30 percent of the land surface of the planet.

What is the big deal? Can't we use the land? Sure. The problem is, because of our gluttony for more and more meat, we are using up the land. God gave us a set amount, and factory farms don't care how much they use. In the United States around 260 million acres of forests have been clear-cut for animals being raised for food.[14]

Our country is not the only culprit. Central America exports approximately 200 million pounds of beef to the United States each year. The land used to raise those cattle comes from clear-cutting forests and rainforests. A Smithsonian study estimates that the necessity for more grazing land means that every minute of every day, a land area equivalent to seven football fields is destroyed in the Amazon Basin.[15]

While destruction of rainforests contributes to land waste, other consequences need to be pondered. Ecological costs include erosion, flooding, and lack of pollination.[17] Furthermore, a ten-kilometer square area of rainforest contains 1,500 various flowering plants and 750 species of trees.[18] Twenty five percent of medicines used in the Western world have been derived from ingredients harvested from these plants in rainforests. Scientists have tested only 1 percent, so we have no idea what is being destroyed.[19]

**Water-Depletion and Pollution**

**Freshwater**

"Now a river went out of Eden to water the garden" (Gn 2:10).

Freshwater resources are a gift of God. We use freshwater to drink, bathe, cook, and irrigate the land—just to name a few. Of all the water resources on earth, 2.5 percent are freshwater. Ocean water accounts for 96.5 percent.[14] More than one billion people in the world do not have the luxury of clean water, and agriculture accounts for 93 percent of water depletion worldwide.[20] Water usage resembles land usage. It is being depleted in a similar way. Crops that feed animals, not humans, have to be watered. Animals have to have drinking water. Water has to be used to cool the CAFOs. If the CAFOs or animals are cleaned, water is used to complete the task.

We are taxing our water supply, but we are also polluting it. One example involves lagoons and sprayfields.

### Lagoons and Sprayfields

Livestock waste contains drug residues, heavy metals, and pathogens. These elements become dangerous if they find their way into our water supply.[21] How do farmers dispose of manure? Two terms of which you should be aware regarding manure management are "lagoons" and "spray fields." Neither of these are safe methods of disposal.

The task of manure management is quite daunting due to sheer volume. For example, a dairy farm that houses 2,500 cows results in a feces and urine production equal to a city of 411,000 people. One of Smithfield Farm's 500,000 hog operations produces enough manure to fill four Yankee Stadiums.[22]

Lagoons are storage ponds typically located near livestock holding areas to allow for easy "scraping" of manure, flush water, urine, wasted feed, etc. into the lagoon for storage. Lagoons hold waste until it is used for land application, or in other words, it is sprayed on crops. Here's where the term "sprayfield" arises.[23]

Lagoons often break or leak or overflow. When this occurs the following contaminants end up in our water supply: nitrogen, phosphorus, pathogens, heavy metals, and microbes. Additionally, because of the conditions in which farmed animals are forced to live, farmers treat them with antibiotics to prevent disease. These antibiotics also end up in the water supply due to such foolish, careless practices. Have you ever heard of antibiotic-resistant strains of bacteria?[24, 25] These bacteria adapt to antibiotics as a result of overuse deeming them no longer effective in humans.

This excerpt from a report by the Natural Resources Defense Council sums up the lagoon's detriment to our clean water well:

"Animal waste also contaminates drinking water supplies. For example, nitrates often seep from lagoons and sprayfields into groundwater. Drinking water contaminated with nitrates can increase the risk of blue baby syndrome, which can cause deaths in infants. High levels of nitrates in drinking water near hog factories have also been linked to spontaneous abortions. Several disease outbreaks related to drinking water have been traced to bacteria and viruses from waste.

On top of this, the widespread use of antibiotics also poses dangers. Large-scale animal factories often give animals antibiotics to promote growth, or to compensate for illness resulting from crowded conditions. These antibiotics are entering the environment and the food chain, contributing to the rise of antibiotic-resistant bacteria and making it harder to treat human diseases."[24]

**My Father's World**

This is God's creation. He gave us power over it. As we are destroying the very place God gave us to live, we are destroying His handiwork: "The heavens declare the glory of God; and the firmament shows His handiwork" (Ps 19:1).

"This is my Father's world,
And to my listening ears
All nature sings, and 'round me rings
The music of the spheres.
This is my Father's world:
I rest me in the thought
Of rocks and trees, of skies and seas
His hand the wonders wrought." (Hymn by Maltbie
Davenport)

Do we believe this hymn? Micah Bennett states in his article, "The Biblical Call to Environmental Stewardship," that "the rampant environmental degradation taking place worldwide today is one of the moral issues most ignored by Christians." What can we do about it?

## A Big Story for a Small Book

As stated at the outset of this chapter, I am no expert in environmental issues. I have barely scratched the surface of this big story. The issues described to you are real and should be addressed. Additionally, while I am a student with you regarding environmentalism, I am aware that our diet makes a huge impact. As a dietitian, I never cease to be amazed at how our food choices affect so much of life—including the environment. As a Christian our good or bad choices affect all of life—including the environment God asked us to steward.

**Take-Home Messages and Tips**

**Limit or Eliminate Animal Products**
As stated in chapter 1, simply cutting meat and animal products from your diet is a huge step in the right direction. Cook meatless meals for your family. At the next potluck dinner, bring a vegetarian meal and share the recipe. Support restaurants that serve vegetarian fare.

**Eat Local**

Supporting local farmers is a great way to eat healthy and support small businesses. Additionally you decrease GHG emissions by limiting transit distance. The food you obtain from local farmers will be fresh and full of nutrients because you also limit the amount of nutrients lost during storage and transit.

**Lead**

Teach those around you about stewarding God's creation. Make other Christians aware of our responsibility. You would be surprised how few people have been exposed to the subject.

**Pray**

Pray that God will help us restore his land.

# Well Said

The insert below was obtained from the group, Climbing for Christ. You can learn about their ministry from: http://www.climbingforchrist.org/Default.aspx?tabid=117

Environmental stewardship is not talk; environmental stewardship is action. Environmental stewardship is practice. Environmental stewardship is practicing the stewardship principles we preach and teach. Stewardship evaluates the consequences of human activity for the household of life; exemplifies Christ's Lordship; is exercised only by human beings; involves accountability to God; is an inescapable condition of human existence; requires freedom to exercise it over a fair share of creation; is exercise of delegated dominion in the service of creation, in which each person is delegated responsibility for all of creation; implies responsibility for and responsibility to; points us to a correct knowledge of our place in things; and is foundational for economics.

*Calvin B. DeWitt is Professor of Environmental Studies at the University of Wisconsin-Madison and is past Director and CEO of Au Sable Institute of Environmental Studies which serves 56 Christian colleges and universities with courses and programs in environmental stewardship in Michigan, Puget Sound, India, and Africa. See Appendix A.*

# Chapter 3

## Human Design

Then God said, "I give you every seed-bearing plant on the face of the whole earth and every tree that has fruit with seed in it. They will be yours for food."

—Genesis 1:29

**Biblical Examples of Our Physiology**

When discussing human physiology, we should begin with the creator of humans. Observations of our original design bring us back to the basics. To accomplish this, we have to go to the beginning of time, to Genesis.

As a Christian, I believe God formed our bodies. We did not evolve from a speck. As evidenced by the following scripture and human anatomy and physiology, i.e., science, we were designed as herbivores. Read below and notice what God gave Adam and Eve to eat.

"Then God said, 'Let us make mankind in our image, in our likeness, so that they may rule over the fish in the sea and the birds in the sky, over the livestock and all the wild animals, and over all the creatures that move along the ground'" Genesis 1:26 .

 "Then God said, 'I give you every seed-bearing plant on the face of the whole earth and every tree that has fruit with seed in it. They will be yours for food.' God saw all that he had made, and it was very good" Genesis 1:29 .

 "Now the Lord God had planted a garden in the east, in Eden; and there he put the man he had formed. The Lord God made all kinds of trees grow out of the ground—trees that were pleasing to the eye and good for food. In the middle of the garden were the tree of life and the tree of the knowledge of good and evil" Genesis 2:8–9.

"The Lord God took the man and put him in the Garden of Eden to work it and take care of it.  And the LORD God commanded the man, 'You are free to eat from any tree in the garden; but you must not eat from the tree of the knowledge of good and evil, for when you eat from it you will certainly die'" Genesis 2:15–17.  Notice that they were not eating animals. In fact, no bloodshed occurred until sin entered the world. God gave them plants to eat.

Now let's look at how God created our bodies by comparing herbivore (plant-eating) and carnivore (meat-eating) anatomy and physiology. Decide to which group we belong. Milton Mills, MD, states, "While most humans are clearly 'behavioral' omnivores (plant and meat eating), the question remains as to whether humans are anatomically suited for a diet that includes animal as well as plant foods."

Carnivores have large claws for tearing flesh. Herbivores have flat, blunt fingertips and nails.

Carnivores have a wide mouth in comparison to their head. They have sharp, pointed teeth, and their saliva does not contain digestive enzymes. Their jaw moves up and down for the most part, not side to side. Herbivore mouth openings are small in comparison to their head. Their teeth are flat and their saliva contains carbohydrate-digesting enzymes. Their jaw moves up and down and side to side.

The carnivore's stomach secretes hydrochloric acid (HCl) keeping the pH level at 1–2, which is needed for protein digestion and killing any bacteria present with rotting flesh foods. Herbivores secrete ten times less HCl. The pH in their stomach is around 4–5, which explains why undercooked meat would make them sick.

A carnivore's small intestine measures three to six times the length of its body. This short length rapidly removes food that will decay. An herbivore's small intestine measures approximately ten to eleven times its body length. This allows for vitamin and mineral absorption from ingested food before transit to the large intestine.

Contrary to what some would like to think, humans are not natural hunters. Every predator that hunts begins in a state of hunger. A starving person does not have the strength to hunt. He or she must eat first.

Think of a lion. This carnivorous animal has a mental state for killing. If a lion sees a small, furry animal, it thinks "attack." Think of a human. Our frame of mind, particularly before the fall was one of compassion, one that reveres life. If we see a furry animal, we want to hold or pet it.

The list could go on. The point I am making is that God's original design of our bodies makes us herbivorous. It makes sense that health follows when humans adopt plant-based diets. A great example of the vitality given when a person eats vegetarian comes from the Book of Daniel. What happens when Daniel refuses the king's food?

"In the third year of the reign of Jehoiakim king of Judah, Nebuchadnezzar king of Babylon came to Jerusalem and besieged it. And the Lord delivered Jehoiakim king of Judah into his hand, along with some of the articles from the temple of God. These he carried off to the temple of his god in Babylonia and put in the treasure house of his god.

Then the king ordered Ashpenaz, chief of his court officials, to bring into the king's service some of the Israelites from the royal family and the nobility—young men without any physical defect, handsome, showing aptitude for every kind of learning, well informed, quick to understand, and qualified to serve in the king's palace. He was to teach them the language and literature of the Babylonians. The king assigned them a daily amount of food and wine from the king's table. They were to be trained for three years, and after that they were to enter the king's service.

Among those who were chosen were some from Judah: Daniel, Hananiah, Mishael, and Azariah. The chief official gave them new names: to Daniel, the name Belteshazzar; to Hananiah, Shadrach; to Mishael, Meshach; and to Azariah, Abednego.

But Daniel resolved not to defile himself with the royal food and wine, and he asked the chief official for permission not to defile himself this way. Now God had caused the official to show favor and compassion to Daniel, but the official told Daniel, "I am afraid of my lord the king, who has assigned your food and drink. Why should he see you looking worse than the other young men your age? The king would then have my head because of you."

Daniel then said to the guard whom the chief official had appointed over Daniel, Hananiah, Mishael, and Azariah, "Please test your servants for ten days: Give us nothing but vegetables to eat and water to drink. Then compare our appearance with that of the young men who eat the royal food, and treat your servants in accordance with what you see." So he agreed to this and tested them for ten days.

"At the end of the ten days they looked healthier and better nourished than any of the young men who ate the royal food. So the guard took away their choice food and the wine they were to drink and gave them vegetables instead." (Dn 1: 1–16)

Enough said. Daniel proves our point precisely.

## Take-Home Messages and Tips

### Think Deeply

Consider Adam and Eve and their utopia in the garden. Consider how God designed their body. They are our original parents. Read the story of Daniel again. Think about the strength he gained eating a plant-based diet.

### Give it a Try

Consult resources provided at the end of the book, and simply try a plant-based diet. See how you feel. If you have never eaten this way, I strongly encourage you to seek help to prevent failure.

### Pray

Pray for direction and wisdom regarding your health and how you might improve.

# Is God Concerned with the Physical Health of Our Bodies?

We have discussed that God created the animals and the environment. He cares about what happens to his creation. He expects us to steward and tend it. God also created our human body, and he cares about it. He expects us to care for it. Finally we are called to glorify God in all we do, including stewarding our health.

**God Cares about Our Health**

I find it comforting that God cares about our health. When one of my children is hurt or sick, God cares. When a loved one is diagnosed with a life-threatening disease, he cares. The life of Jesus reveals this time and again.

He has compassion on our weaknesses. He heals us.

"[It is God] who forgives all your sins and heals all your diseases, who redeems your life from the pit and crowns you with love and compassion" (Ps 103:3–4).

"When Jesus saw him lying there and learned that he had been in this condition for a long time, he asked him, 'Do you want to get well?' 'Sir,' the invalid replied, 'I have no one to help me into the pool when the water is stirred. While I am trying to get in, someone else goes down ahead of me.' Then Jesus said to him, 'Get up! Pick up your mat and walk.' At once the man was cured; he picked up his mat and walked" (Jn 5:6–8).

## God Calls Us to Care for Our Bodies

In Romans 12, Paul asserts that presenting our body as a living sacrifice acceptable to God is our "reasonable" service. "Reasonable" is the way the service is described. He did not refer to service as an over-the-top kind of action. It is just plain reasonable.

Again Paul states in Ephesians 5:28–30, "In this same way, husbands ought to love their wives as their own bodies. He who loves his wife loves himself. After all, no one ever hated their own body, but they feed and care for their body, just as Christ does the church." Paul takes it for granted that people care for their own body.

In 1 Corinthians 6:19, you read, "Do you not know that your bodies are temples of the Holy Spirit, who is in you, whom you have received from God? You are not your own." This passage is similar to one you find about Solomon: if you were called to build a temple for God, would you go to the lengths that he did? In 1 Kings 6:20, read that Solomon "overlaid the inside with pure gold, and he also overlaid the altar of cedar." Solomon used the best resources. He did not cut corners for his Lord. 1 Corinthians tells us we house God now. What kind of temple does he have in us? What resources are you using to build his home in your body?

## Glorifying God

"So whether you eat or drink or whatever you do, do it all for the glory of God." Glorifying God with our health may seem secondary to other spiritual disciplines. However, in the words of Dr. Kenneth H. Cooper referring to Christians, "They fail to understand that their spiritual lives— including values and relationships that they hold dear— are closely connected with the conditions of their bodies. If the body begins to break down, the person may lack the endurance and energy required to serve others, stay in a good mood, or even spend extended times in prayer...And worst of all, your service for the Lord will suffer if your health begins to break down."

## Final Thoughts

Evidence should be mounting in your mind that glorifying God with our diet is more complicated in today's world. In the midst of the confusion, simplicity can be the answer. Eat as close to nature as possible. God is the author of nature. Eat food that grows from the ground, which is God's original design before the fall. Stay away from processed food. If you choose to eat meat, avoid animals that have been abused and polluted. Meat avoidance triumphs as the more beneficial choice. The following chapters explain why.

# Chapter 4

## But We Need Animals for Food. Right? Wrong.

As soon as I realized that I didn't need meat to survive or to be in good health, I began to see how forlorn it all is. If only we had a different mentality about the drama of the cowboy and the range and all the rest of it. It's a very romantic notion, an entrenched part of American culture, but I've seen, for example, pigs waiting to be slaughtered, and their hysteria and panic was something I shall never forget.

—Cloris Leachman

## Caring for Our Bodies, Minus Animals

Animal products are not necessary or helpful for a healthy diet. As a caveat, I acknowledge that there are numerous food products that are not meat based and that lead to poor health: sugar, artificial ingredients, preservatives, and so on. For our purposes, the focus will remain on animal products. This chapter exposes why you may think you need animal products in your diet. In turn it reveals the truth about why you do not. As today's Christian, we have to look at the food industry, and "therefore, be shrewd as snakes" (Mt 10:16). We have to find the truth and transform our minds.

## Vegetarian Does Not Equal Deficiency

At the mention of vegetarian nutrition, immediately people begin to think "deficiency." How many times have I been asked the questions: where would I get protein? Don't I need milk for strong bones? Won't I be malnourished if I don't eat meat? Questions like these come from advertising and marketing. You have been told you need these products. It is no different than any other marketed product. Bounty paper towels work better than the leading brand for spills we are told. Allstate tells us we are in good hands if they insure us, and choosy moms choose Jiff. Think back further. You deserve a break today—McDonalds. Tastes great-less filling—Miller Lite. The list could go on and on. These messages stick with us though. We begin to feel we need the advertised items. Advertising for meat and milk is no different, just darker. Milk—"it does a body good." Beef—"it's what's for dinner." Pork—it's "the other white meat."

## This Advertising Is Darker—Milk.

Our government actually participates in this advertising. Why? Money. Take the dairy industry as an example. The dairy industry has incredible political spending power that actually doubled between 1998 and 2008. Contributions of 4.8 million dairy industry dollars were awarded to federal candidates in the 2008 election cycle.[4] See Table 1 for contribution information in 2011–2012. Is it any wonder that our government assists these groups in their marketing strategies? For example, the United States Department of Agriculture (USDA) administers the "Got Milk" campaign.[5]

*Source: Center for Responsive Politics(Open Secrets.org)

**The bold, underlined companies are related to meat and dairy.

## TABLE 1. Top Contributors, 2011–2012 Presidential Election

| Contributor | Amount |
|---|---|
| American Crystal Sugar | $956,500 |
| Altria Group | $647,270 |
| Weaver Popcorn | $334,900 |
| Farm Credit Council | $285,095 |
| Publix Super Markets | $276,900 |
| **California Dairies Inc**. | $274,400 |
| American Veterinary Medical Assn. | $217,500 |
| International Paper | $199,676 |
| Flo-Sun Inc. | $189,040 |
| **Monsanto Co** | $164,500 |
| Swisher International | $161,000 |
| Reynolds American | $158,075 |
| Weyerhaeuser Co. | $152,050 |
| **Dean Foods** | $150,750 |
| **Smithfield Foods** | $142,442 |
| **National Cattlemen's Beef Assn** | $141,219 |
| **American Farm Bureau** | $122,546 |
| American Sugar Cane League | $122,000 |
| **Kraft Foods** | $121,984 |
| Minn-Dak Farmers Co-Op | $102,500 |

# Compliments of Center for Responsive Politics ** April 2010

The dairy industry includes dairy farmers, cheese and butter manufacturers, ice cream producers, and makers of other dairy-related products. The industry's political spending power has steadily increased over the past decade, resulting in contributions more than doubling between 1998 and 2008.

The industry contributed $4.8 million to federal candidates during the 2008 election cycle, with 60 percent going to Republicans. The top contributor was the Dairy Farmers of America (DFA), a dairy farmers' cooperative. People and political action committees associated with the DFA contributed $925,000 to federal candidates, with 53 percent going to Democrats. Other top contributors include dairy manufacturers such as California Dairies Inc., Dean Foods, and Land O'Lakes.

In addition, the industry spent $4.7 million on federal lobbying efforts in 2009—near a historic high set in 2007. Trade associations and dairy cooperates are by far the biggest industry spenders when it comes to lobbying. The DFA and its subsidiaries spent more than $860,000 in 2009, while the International Dairy Foods Association and National Milk Producers Federation each spent well into the six-figure range.

Like much of the agriculture sector, the dairy industry historically has contributed more money to Republicans, giving them 60 percent of total contributions during the past two decades.

However, who receives the dairy industry's money also depends heavily on which political party is in power.

After losing Congress in 1994, the percentage of contributions Democrats received plummeted from 61 percent to 32 percent in just two years. After retaking Congress in 2006 and making more gains in 2008, that percentage has climbed from 29 percent in 2006 to 54 percent midway through the 2010 election cycle.

Issues important to the industry include health and safety regulations, environmental concerns—particularly regarding air and water standards—and international trade issues such as import quotas that protect its business.

Of recent concern to the dairy industry has been how, if at all, their greenhouse gas emissions will be regulated under any proposed federal cap-and-trade legislation, or by the Environmental Protection Agency.

This has led the industry into uncharted territory. For example, the political action committee of California Dairies Inc. contributed $10,000 to the 2010 campaign of Sen. Lisa Murkowski (R-Alaska), the first contribution to her campaign from a dairy producer. It is likely not a coincidence that Murkowski is the ranking member on the Senate Energy and Natural Resources Committee, and a vocal opponent of the EPA regulating greenhouse gases.

## Young Targets

The milk industry's advertising targets Americans at an early age. My children reported in the past (kindergarten through third grade so far) learning about healthy eating by the Food Guide Pyramid in their public school. The now outdated USDA Food Guide Pyramid recommended that Americans drink three glasses of milk daily. The USDA also untruthfully boasted that the pyramid is intended for the majority of Americans.[1] The majority of Americans are lactose intolerant (i.e., milk makes them sick). See figures below.[2]

## Figure 1: Food Guide Pyramid

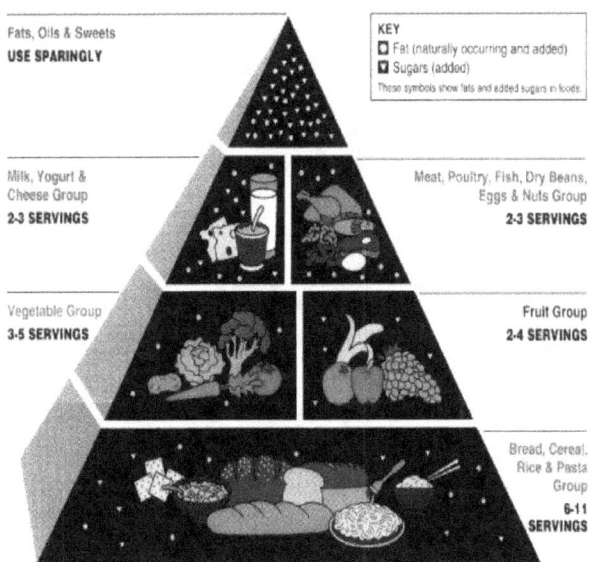

My Plate replaced the pyramid and still portrays milk as a necessity.

Figure 2: My Plate

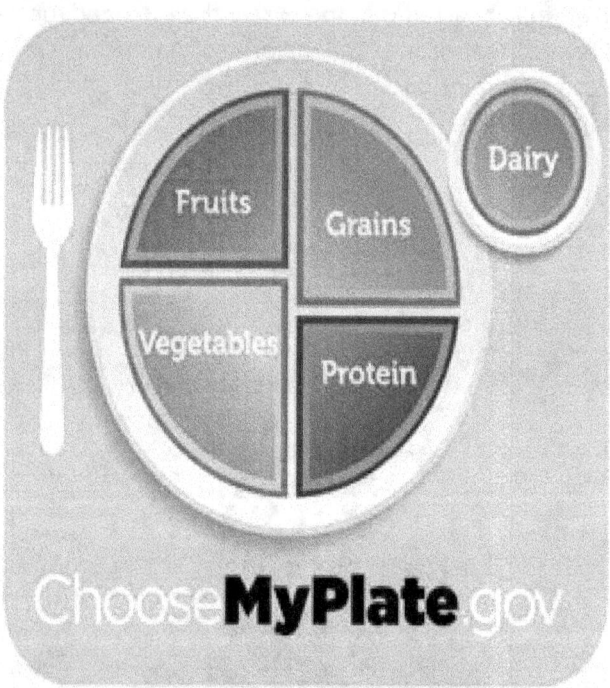

Harvard School of Public Health developed a more evidence-based My Plate.

## Figure 3: Harvard Healthy Eating Plate

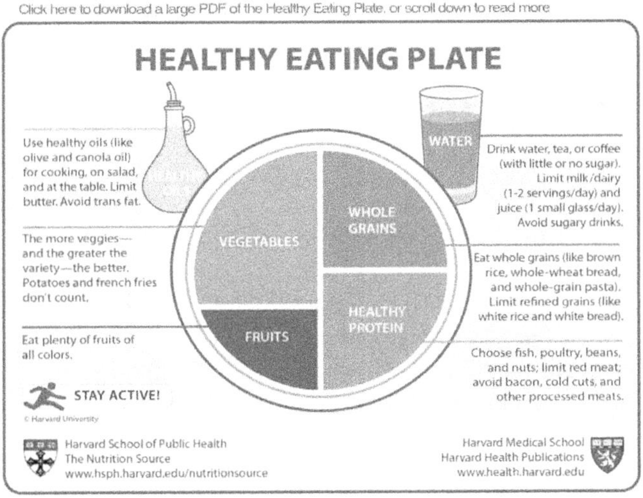

The daily milk requirement our government recommends is not grounded on evidenced-based research. That presents a real problem to me. I would go so far as to call it false advertising.

**Advertising through Feeding the Vulnerable**

The story gets more complicated. After advertising in the traditional sense and educating students in school, the government actually buys these products. Our government disguises the purchases with the words "food subsidies." Our taxes then pay for them as part of programs such as The National School Lunch Program; the Special Supplemental Nutrition Program for Women; Women, Infants and Children (WIC); and the Emergency Food Assistance Program, which targets women, children, and the poor. The United States government has enormous purchasing power. Thus it can buy food and sell it to these programs at a cheap rate. Translation: your and my tax dollars are paying for this food whether we eat it or not. Additionally, the subsidies are fed to vulnerable groups like children and low-income women. The percentages of foods purchased by the United States government in 2006–2007 are as follows:[3]

- Meat—3 percent

- Poultry and eggs—15 percent

- Cheese—22 percent

- Fruits and vegetables—25 percent (35 percent of these are potatoes)

- Grains, peanuts, and oils—3 percent

So, the government advertises for dairy and then forces taxpayers to buy it. Provision of these foods to such worthy programs sends a message to participants: they are necessary for good health. Let's return to the public school system to see what messages the parents, teachers, and students receive.

**Nutrition Education in Public Schools**

Our government's Special Milk Program teaches parents and children that milk is necessary for good health. Institutions that participate in the program provide their milk on a nonprofit basis and in return receive reimbursement from our government. In 2009, this program cost $14 million with over 78 million pints of milk served. The program has expanded to the National School Lunch and School Breakfast Programs.[6] When children in our public school systems purchase a lunch tray, you can be sure that it will include milk according to the Richard B.

**Russell National School Lunch Act (amended July 2, 2004). See below.**

Sec.9 (2) FLUID MILK -

A. IN GENERAL.—Lunches served by schools participating in the school lunch program under this Act:

i. shall offer students fluid milk in a variety of fat contents;

ii. may offer students flavored and unflavored fluid milk and lactose-free fluid milk; and

iii. shall provide a substitute for fluid milk for students whose disability restricts their diet, on receipt of a written statement from a licensed physician that identifies the disability that restricts the student's diet and that specifies the substitute for fluid milk.

B. RESTRICTIONS ON SALE OF MILK PROHIBITED. A school that participates in the school lunch program under this Act shall not directly or indirectly restrict the sale or marketing of fluid milk products by the school (or a person approved by the school) at any time or any place."[7]

### What Is My Problem?

My problem is this. Parents come to me wanting to know what to feed their children. Government programs and education create confusion for well-meaning parents because of the almighty dollar. Women with low incomes are given milk to feed their children. Women are mistakenly eating cheese and drinking milk to "strengthen" their bones, finding out despite their efforts they have osteoporosis.

Let me appeal to your common sense and also give you science to help you understand my frustration.

## Common Sense—Digestibility of Dairy

Can it really be that the USDA Food Guide Pyramid and My Plate are for the majority of Americans? Has the USDA looked around at Americans lately? I have, and I see many colors of skin and a variety of ethnicities. The USDA requires milk be served on the trays of American children. The problem? Most of these children are lactose intolerant, especially children of color. Why would we put milk in front of them to drink daily at school? Why would we offer milk to less fortunate children as a supposedly helpful program?

Examine this table to see just how many groups are lactose intolerant.

## TABLE 1.[8] Lactose Intolerance and Ethnicity

| Ethnic groups that are 60–100 percent lactose intolerant: |
| --- |
| Near East and Mediterranean: Arabs, Ashkenazi Jews, Greek Cypriots, Southern Italians |
| Asia: Thais, Indonesians, Chinese, Koreans |
| Africa: South Nigerians, Hausa, Bantu |
| North and South America: black Americans, Latinos, Eskimos, Canadian and American Indians, Chami Indians |
| Ethnic groups that are 2–30 percent lactose intolerant: |
| Northern Europeans |
| Africa: Himu, Tussi, Nomadic Fulani |
| India: Individuals from Punjab and New Delhi |

I have a hard time believing it is ethical or Christ-like to place on children's trays items that will harm them. The dairy industry could care less and would appreciate parents remaining in the dark on the matter. Enlightenment comes through using common sense.

## Common Sense—Milk throughout the Life Cycle—Is It Needed?

Has it ever crossed your mind that humans are the only species on the planet that drink the milk of a different species? Ask yourself why we chose the cow? Why not drink elephant milk or giraffe milk? Mark Hyman wrote in the *Huffington Post* in 2010 that "dairy is nature's perfect food—but only if you're a calf." Calves even stop drinking their mother's milk once they are weaned!

If that's the case, why are we made to feel we must give our children milk for strong bones and growth? The answer includes hidden truths, false advertising, and lack of education.

### Milk Babies

"Perhaps when the public is educated as to the hazards of milk, only calves will be left to drink the real thing." (Frank Oski, MD, former professor of pediatrics, Johns Hopkins University School of Medicine; past president, United States Society for Pediatric Research.)

### Nutrients in Milk—The Truth

God designed the nutrient content of each species' milk to be absolutely perfect to meet the needs of its babies. Check out the following tables that illustrate this point. They depict the nutritional breakdown of different species milk. Each one differs to support the growth needs of that particular animal.

**TABLE 2. Comparison of Milk from Differing Species**

|  | Protein | Carbohydrate | Sodium | Phosphorus | Calcium |
|---|---|---|---|---|---|
| Human | 1.1 | 9 | 16 | 18 | 33 |
| Cow | 4 | 4.9 | 50 | 97 | 118 |

**TABLE 3. Milk Sources and Protein**

| Milk Source | Percent of Calories as Protein | Number of Days in which Birth Weight Doubles. |
|---|---|---|
| Human | 5 | 180 |
| Horse | 11 | 60 |
| Cow | 15 | 47 |
| Goat | 17 | 19 |
| Dog | 30 | 8 |
| Cat | 40 | 7 |
| Rat | 49 | 4 |

**Source: Joseph Keon, *WhiteWash: The Disturbing Truth About Cow's Milk and Your Health*.

Notice the vast difference in protein levels and how long for birth weight to double between human and cow milk. Do you find it odd that Americans think it's a good idea to feed their infants the milk of a cow? In actuality a horse would more closely resemble human milk.

**Breast Milk—The Obvious Right Choice**

Of course breast milk represents the most nutritious food source for our babies. I am not one to make mothers who love their babies feel like demons if they can't breast-feed. Some struggle so much that the whole process ruins their joy of being a mom. There are many facets of motherhood, and many wonderful moms did not breast-feed. However, is breast-feeding best for the baby? Absolutely. In fact, as a dietitian, it is the only choice I am comfortable recommending.

**More Common Sense Regarding Bones**

Older Children—Science Refutes the "Requirement" for Cow's Milk

Our government claims a calcium crisis is placing our children at risk for poor bone health. This crisis sends Americans down the path of needing to provide more milk for their children.[9, 10]We are dealing with more false advertising. Research doesn't support this milk solution. In fact, the Federal Trade Commission actually requested that the USDA show scientific proof regarding their milk-mustache campaigns after a panel of scientists drew opposing conclusions. One opposing conclusion determined that no compelling evidence exists linking dairy to strong bones.[11, 12]

Lanou and colleagues conducted a meta-analysis (compilation and review) of thirty-seven studies regarding dairy and supplemental calcium. Of the thirty-seven studies, twenty-seven showed no relationship between dairy or supplemental calcium and bone mineralization/fracture risk in children and adolescents.[13]

A study involving female teen exercise patterns was performed. In this study, calcium showed no relation to

BMD at eighteen years of age or bone mineral gain from twelve to eighteen years of age. Exercise did improve BMD and mineral gain.[14]

The late, well-known pediatrician Dr. Benjamin Spock had this to say about dairy:

> "Thanks in part to clever and persuasive advertising, everyone knows that milk is an important source of calcium. But among themselves, scientists debate the pluses and minuses of cow's milk when it comes to bone health. For example, several well-done studies found no connection between the amount of cow's milk children drink and the amount of calcium they store in their bones. That is really a remarkable finding. If drinking cow's milk is important for bone growth, then you'd expect that people who drink more milk would have stronger bones. But they don't. In fact, the United States has very high per capita milk consumption and also very high rates of osteoporosis."[15]

Not only does research not support dairy for bone mineralization in children, research points out that dairy poses threats to other aspects of children's health.

**Health Risks of Milk in Children**

The jury is still out, but many studies are linking early feeding of cow's milk to type 1 diabetes. While type 1 diabetes is an autoimmune disease involving genetics, it also develops partially due to environmental triggers. One of the observed triggers is an immune reaction to cow milk protein. This is evidenced by increased antibodies to milk proteins found in type 1 diabetics. A meta-analysis of twenty well designed studies concluded statistically significant associations between early introduction of cow milk and type 1 diabetes.[16, 17, 18]

Milk presents more health risks to children. Dr. Spock continues:

> "Milk is the number one source of fat in children's diet in the Unites States—higher than burgers, fries, and chips. (A cup of whole milk has 4.6 grams of saturated fat, more than 4 slices of bacon; a tablespoon of butter has 7.3 grams.) Doctors recommend whole milk for toddlers from age one to two because the brain is growing rapidly then. But the omega 3 fatty acids that are also essential for brain development are found in vegetable oils; cow's milk is very low in these healthy fats...Dairy food can impair a child's ability to absorb iron, and can cause blood loss from the intestines in small children and in children who are allergic to cow's milk...Allergic reactions to proteins in cow's milk are common. If asthma or eczema runs in the family, there's a good chance that milk might be a contributing cause...A sensitivity to cow's milk sometimes triggers constipation, ear infections, and even (in rare cases) type 1 diabetes."[14]

If milk does not benefit children the way we have been led to believe, what about the other common target population—women?

## Dairy for Women—Dispelling the Osteoporosis Lie

Again, I refer to Harvard School of Public Health and their views on governmental dairy nutritional guidelines:

"The guidelines' recommendation to increase the intake of low-fat milk and dairy products seems to reflect the interests of the powerful dairy industry more so than the latest science. There is little, if any, evidence that eating dairy prevents osteoporosis or fractures, and there is considerable evidence that high dairy product consumption is associated with increased risk of fatal prostate and maybe ovarian cancers."[19]

A twelve-year prospective study focused on milk and dietary sources of calcium. The purpose was to scrutinize the validity of public-health messages that advise increased milk consumption for osteoporosis prevention. The population studied included 77,761 female nurses aged thirty-five to fifty-nine at baseline in 1980. In this cohort, women who consumed larger amounts of calcium from dairy had modest, but statistically significant increased risks for hip fracture. Women who consumed calcium from nondairy sources showed no increase in fracture risk.[20]

How can this be? Milk comforts. Americans believe in milk. Advertising sells.

If dairy doesn't grow children's bones or protect adult's bones what does? Calcium and vitamin D are structural components of bone, but there is more to the story.

## Calcium

There are two areas to consider regarding calcium:
absorption rates of food and preventing loss.

### Absorption

How much calcium do we actually absorb from milk versus
other sources? Table 4 reveals the level of absorption.[9]

**TABLE 4. Calcium Absorption Rates**

| Food | Serving Size (in cups) | Calcium/ Serving | Calcium Absorbed/Serving | Amount Needed to Absorb 100 mg Calcium (in cups) |
|---|---|---|---|---|
| Orange Juice- Calcium Fortified | 1 | 300 | 108 | 7/8 |
| 2% Milk | 1 | 297 | 95 | 1 |
| Soy Milk- Calcium Fortified | 1 | 300 | 93 | 1 |
| Mixed Grain Cereal | 1 | 306 | 92 | 1 |
| Kale, Frozen | ½ | 90 | 53 | 1 |
| Turnip Greens, Frozen | ½ | 99 | 51 | 1 |

When compared with cow's milk, one cup of kale, turnip
greens, soy milk, and cereal are absorbed just as well.
Fortified orange juice fares slightly better. These values
disprove the "requirement" of cow's milk as a calcium
source.

## Preventing Loss

The issue with milk's lack of bone-protection capabilities involves the animal protein content. What happens to our bones when humans eat animal protein?

It appears that the higher the intake of animal protein, the weaker the bones. A study evaluated dietary intake of 1,035 women through food-frequency questionnaires. Researchers controlled for other factors that would cause bone loss such as weight, estrogen use, tobacco use, exercise, etc. The women were categorized into three groups: high ratio of animal to vegetable protein, middle ratio of animal to vegetable protein, and low ratio of animal to vegetable protein. They then took the ratios to compare BMD, bone loss, and fractures in a seven-year follow-up. The initial BMD was the same in all groups. The high-ratio group had three times the bone loss and 3.7 times the rate of hip fractures of the low ratio group.[21] Why is this?

Every food we digest produces an "ash": acid or base. Animal protein produces an acid ash. Vegetables produce higher levels of base. Our bodies achieve pH balance by excreting excess acid in the urine. As we age, we become less efficient at the process so we need a buffer. Calcium is base, i.e., a buffer. Bone is our reservoir of calcium. When women eat diets high in animal protein, the blood needs to be buffered due to the acidity caused by diet. Bone resorption (breakdown) accomplishes this by the transfer of calcium from bones to the blood. High meat and dairy intake, therefore equals weak bones.

Why don't we hear this more often? The answer is false advertising and truth suppression. We are told dairy intake yields strong bones. We are told we need meat.

## Truth Telling Regarding Meat

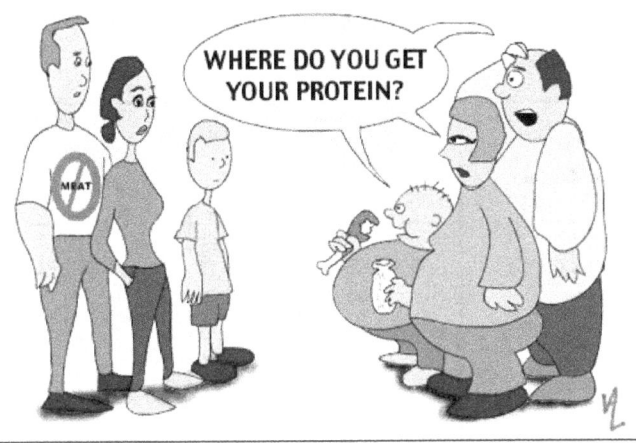

Latest studies: A third of Americans are overweight, and an additional quarter are obese.

Source: http://living-vegan.blogspot.com/2007/03/where-do-you-get-your-protein.html.

The above cartoon represents a never-ending question and running joke among those who eat a plant-based diet. Let's look again at the American population. How many protein-malnourished people do you see walking around? I see them on television commercials involving impoverished children. I even see them in hospitals and dialysis centers, but never in the healthy population. On the other hand, there are many people who are well fed, obese, and undernourished in vitamins and minerals. Table 5 displays a portion of the dietary reference intake chart—what our government recommends to prevent protein deficiency.

## TABLE 5.[22] Governmental Recommendations Regarding Protein Intake

| Dietary Reference Intakes: Macronutrients Nutrient | Life Stage Group (in years) | RDA/AI* g/d [a] |
|---|---|---|
| Protein and amino acids | Infants | 9.1* |
| | 0–6 months | 11.0 |
| | 7–12 months | 13 |
| | Children | 19 |
| | 1–3 | 34 |
| | 4–8 | 52 |
| | Males | 56 |
| | 9–13 | 56 |
| | 14–18 | 56 |
| | 19–30 | 56 |
| | 31–50 | 34 |
| | 50–70 | 46 |
| | > 70 | 46 |
| | Females | 46 |
| | 9–13 | 46 |
| | 14–18 | 46 |
| | 19–30 | 71 |
| | 31–50 | 71 |
| | 50–70 | 71 |
| | > 70 | 71 |
| | Pregnancy | 71 |
| | ≤ 18 | 71 |
| | 19–30 | |
| | 31–50 | |
| | Lactation | |
| | ≤ 18 | |
| | 19–30 | |
| | 31–50 | |

*DRI-Dietary Reference Intakes-Basic guidelines for daily intake of nutrients. Includes RDA and AI.

*RDA- Recommended Daily Allowance-Essentially replaced by DRI. Historically referred to the nutrient level needed to meet 97-98% of the population for a particular gender and age group.

*AI-Adequate Intake-Sets an appropriate level of intake when scientific data are insufficient to establish an actual requirement.

Now look at the following two samples of one-day menus. They are merely samples, but not far from reality. People assume their diet is deficient when the diet lacks meat. However, notice the enormous amount of protein provided in the typical American menu. Compare it to the recommended daily allowance (RDA) listed above. The typical American diet supplies way more than the RDA. The plant-based diet is much closer to the RDA for protein. Notice the differences in provision of vitamins and minerals. The plant-based diet is much more abundant in these items. In fact, the only shortage displayed with a whole food, plant-based diet is that of fat, calories, and likely sodium. This is a bonus.

| Typical American Menu | Plant-Based Menu |
| --- | --- |
| **Breakfast:** | **Breakfast:** |
| 2 Eggs | 1 C Oatmeal |
| 2 Slices Bacon | 2 Toast, 1 T Vegan Spread, |
| 2 T All Fruit | |
| 2 Toast, 1 T Butter, 2 T Jelly | 1 C Strawberries |
| 1 C Coffee | 1 C Coffee |
| | |
| **Lunch:** | **Lunch:** |
| Fast Food Cheeseburger | Veggie Burger |
| Medium Fry | 1 Bowl Lentil Soup |
| Large Diet Coke | 1 Glass Tea |
| | |
| **Dinner:** | **Dinner:** |
| 1 Chicken Breast | 1 C Black Beans |
| 1 C Potatoes | 1 C Broccoli |
| 1 C Green Beans | 1 C Squash |
| 1 Roll | 1 Whole Wheat Roll |
| Water | Water |
| | |
| **Snack:** | **Snack:** |
| 1 Bag Doritos | Handful Almonds |
| Apple | Apple |

## Table 6: Nutrient Breakdown of Opposing Menus

| Nutrients | Typical American Menu | Plant-Based Menu |
|---|---|---|
| Calories (Kcal) | 2688 | 1455 |
| Fat (g) | 149 | 51 |
| Protein (g) | 148 | 69 |
| Carbohydrate (g) | 347 | 224 |
| Fiber (g) | 25 | 55 |
| Sodium (mg) | 4598 | 1523 |
| Calcium (mg) | 774 | 611 |
| Vitamin D (IU) | 144 | 200 |
| Vitamin A (IU) | 3277 | 6127 |
| Vitamin C (mg) | 43 | 227 |
| Folate | 342 | 594 |

**Values taken from USDA nutrient database or manufacturer.

**Most food sources of vitamin D come from fortification. Eggs were the major source in the typical American menu and a smart balance (brand of buttery spread I recommend that does not contain trans-fats. I choose the light version) in the plant-based menu.

A plant-based diet will improve your health immensely by providing abundant vitamins and minerals. Animal-based foods provide cholesterol and fat. They are lacking in fiber, vitamins, and minerals, making them unnecessary.

**Take-Home Messages and Tips**

**Calcium**
Review the sources of calcium provided in this chapter, and include them in your diet.

**Vitamin D**

Vitamin D comes from the sun. Spending ten to fifteen minutes a day two to three times a week in the sunlight will help. Orange juice and alternative milks such as almond milk are often fortified with vitamin D.

**Bone Protection**

Animal protein weakens bones. Remove it from your diet, or a t the very least, investigate ways to cut back.

**Breast-Feed**

God designed human breast milk especially for human babies. If you struggle with the process, contact a lactation consultant. Do the best you can.

**Listen to Research**

When learning about your body and health, look at information that has been researched. Be careful to find out who or what group performed the research. Did they have financial ties?

# Chapter 5

## Acute Danger by Meat

Nothing will benefit human health and increase chances for survival of life on earth as much as the evolution to a vegetarian diet.

—Albert Einstein

**Quick Review**

We have discussed CAFOs and the harm imposed on animals and the environment. Chapter 3 skimmed the surface of the injury animal products inflict on our human health. Let's delve further into the reason animal products are not beneficial: their impact on human health.

Illness can be classified in two ways: acute and chronic. Acute illness has a rapid onset and will be resolved quickly or can be deadly. Chronic illness typically develops more slowly and may be cured or last a person's lifespan. Examples of chronic illness include cancer and heart disease. They will be discussed in chapters 5 and 6. Diets involving animal protein contribute to these illnesses. Let's begin with an examination of acute illness.

**The Quick and Deadly Onset of *E. coli* 0157:H7**

*E. coli* 0157:H7 is a bacterium found in contaminated water and food. Hamburger meat represents a common reservoir of the bacteria, thus explaining why *E. coli* is referred to as the "hamburger disease." When ingested, *E. coli* 0157:H7 secretes toxins in the human intestinal tract causing gastrointestinal (GI) upset, which is characterized by bloody diarrhea.

In the worst cases, *E. coli* 0157:H7 causes death. Unfortunately, the weaker citizens of our society, children and the elderly, are the casualties of *E. coli* 0157:H7.

Why do some who are infected with *E. coli* 0157:H7 live and others do not? Some develop hemolytic-uremia syndrome (HUS), typified by hemolytic anemia, thrombocytopenia, and renal failure. This condition advances most commonly in our vulnerable populations.[6] Around 15 percent of *E. coli* 0157:H7-infected children acquire HUS.[7] As a whole, an estimated 10 percent of people diseased with *E. coli* 0157:H7 contract HUS. Of those, despite heroic efforts by medical personnel, 10 percent will die.[5]

**Kids like Lauren and Kevin**

"For I tell you that their angels in heaven always see the face of my Father in heaven" (Mt 18:10).

Do you remember the situation that happened at Jack in the Box in 1992? It was November 1992 through February 1993 when Jack in the Box issued a recall on all ground beef still in the restaurants due to an outbreak of *E. coli* O157:H7. More than seven hundred people across four states became ill. Two hundred were hospitalized. Who was hurt the most? Children were and four died. One of those victims was a little girl by the name of Lauren Beth Rudolph. On Christmas Eve, 1992, she was admitted to the hospital with extreme pain. Through the course of her illness, she suffered three heart attacks. She died on December 28, 1992, at age six while her mother held her.[1,2]

Another case of contamination with *E. coli* O157:H7 was recorded in 2001. The victim's name was Kevin. He was a perfectly healthy little two-and-a-half-year-old boy. That year he and his parents unknowingly had burgers that were contaminated with *E. coli* O157:H7. Twelve days later he was dead.[3]

Children are more prone to be affected by *E. coli* 0157:H7 for several reasons:

- Their immune systems are still developing thus the ability to fight infection is hindered.
- They have less body mass so the dose of the pathogen required to sicken them is less.
- Their stomachs produce less acid so their capacity to kill harmful bacteria is diminished.[4]

## Elderly

"Do not cast me away when I am old; do not forsake me when my strength is gone" (Ps 71:9).

One of the largest *E. coli* 0157:H7 outbreaks occurred in Scotland from December 1996 through January 1997. More than four hundred people were infected from contaminated beef. Twenty of those, the majority of which were elderly citizens who attended a church luncheon for retirees in Wishaw, died.[5]

## Isolated Events?

While these events were highlighted in an effort to put a face to the tragedy of *E. coli* 0157:H7, these events are not isolated. The following outline of investigations by the Centers for Disease Control into *E. coli* 0157:H7 outbreaks proves this.

## E. coli Outbreak Investigations[8]

2011
- Multistate Outbreak of *E. coli* O157:H7 Infections Linked to Romaine Lettuce
- Outbreak of Shiga toxin-producing *E. coli* O104 (STEC O104:H4) Infections Associated with Travel to Germany
- Multistate Outbreak of *E. coli* O157:H7 Infections Associated with Lebanon Bologna
- Multistate Outbreak of *E. coli* O157:H7 Infections Associated with In-shell Hazelnuts

2010
- Bravo Farms Cheeses - *E. coli* O157:H7
- Shredded Romaine Lettuce from a Single Processing Facility - *E. coli* O145
- Infections Associated with Beef from National Steak and Poultry - *E. coli* O157:H7

2009
- Beef from Fairbank Farms - *E. coli* O157:H7
- Beef from JBS Swift Beef Company - *E. coli* O157:H7
- Prepackaged Cookie Dough - *E. coli* O157:H7

2008
- Beef from Kroger/Nebraska Ltd - *E. coli* O157:H7

2007
- Totino's/Jeno's Pizza - *E. coli* O157:H7
- Topp's Ground Beef Patties - *E. coli* O157:H7

2006
- Fresh Spinach - *E. coli* O157:H7

## Contributions of the Meat Industry to *E. coli* 0157:H7

The meat industry contributes to our risk of ingesting *E. coli* O157:H7 in several ways: through feeding and slaughter of animals, and pollution.

### Feeding

God didn't design cows to eat corn. Cows naturally eat grass. Feeding cows corn began after World War II. Common practice was that cows were fed grass until a few months prior to slaughter at which point some corn was mixed into their feed. Corn increased the amount of fat and marbling in the meat.[9] It turns out, however, that feeding corn to cows is not a good idea. In the words of John Robbins,

> "Feeding grain to cattle has got to be one of the dumbest ideas in the history of Western civilization...When cattle are fed corn, their gastrointestinal tracts become acidic. Acidic environments promote the E. coli bacteria. While cattle farmers may produce fattened cows faster to make a buck and supposedly 'save the environment', E. coli 0157:H7 kills people who eat undercooked hamburger."[10]

When cows ate grass, they had a more neutral-pH environment in their gut. When we then ate the beef, the microbes that had lived in the cows' guts died in our more acidic gut. Once cows started to be fed on corn, everything changed. Their pH became closer to ours, and *E. coli* adapted to live in more acidic environments. As a result, *E. coli* 0157:H7 can now live in our gut. CAFOs continue to use corn anyway.

## Slaughter

In the 1950s, cows lived four to five years before going to slaughter. Today cows are ready for kill at fourteen to sixteen months thanks to corn feeding. More cows slaughtered equals more money made.[10]

The way that animals are slaughtered adds to the problem. Due to the sloppy, fast-paced nature of modern slaughter, fecal matter ends up in packaged meat. Fecal matter of corn-fed cows has high levels of *E. coli* 0157:H7. In simpler terms, there is poo in the meat, and poo houses *E. coli* 0157:H7.

## Pollution

Remember lagoons and sprayfields discussed in chapter 2? Spraying this fecal matter onto vegetables puts those of us who don't eat meat at risk. Lagoons that spill into the water supply used for irrigation also contaminate vegetables. An example is the 2006 recall of spinach due to *E. coli* 0157:H7.[11]

## Ethical Solutions?

God has a design for a purpose. If cows lived the way God had designed, they would be in the open eating grass. Without CAFOs, fewer cows would be raised. There would be less manure. The manure would fertilize the grass that the cows would eat. Less manure would end up in our water supply. We would have less if any *E. coli* 0157:H7.

## CAFO Solutions?

The meat industry decided that instead of conducting farming in an ethical, God honoring way, they would continue shady feeding practices and animal confinement. The solution to animal illness and death caused by these techniques led the industry to blend low doses of antibiotics into animal feed and water. These antibiotics also help promote faster growth. Have you ever heard the phrase "antibiotic-resistant strains of bacteria"? This is yet another contribution of CAFOs. Methicillin-resistant staphylococcus aureus (MRSA) is an example of an acute illness resulting from antibiotic resistance.

## Personal Experience with MRSA

When working at a dialysis center, I remember asking one of our nurses why she was putting red dots on some of the patients' flow sheets. She whispered to me, "MRSA." This was in 2008. I had been working in dialysis since 1997 and had never before seen that.

I left dialysis to work on a quality-improvement project for Medicare. During this time a friend said her son had a spider bite and she would be taking him to the pediatrician. She later reported it was no spider bite. It turned out to be MRSA. She acquired it also. Thankfully none of the people I knew got seriously ill or died, but where was it all coming from? MRSA used to be an infection seen mainly in hospitals.

## Pig Farms

Khanna and colleagues conducted a study in 2007 where they investigated twenty Ontario, Canada, farms. Forty-five percent of the 285 pigs studied had MRSA. This study also supported the concern regarding the transfer of MRSA from pigs to humans.[12] Though an estimated nine million Canadian hogs were imported to the United States that year, the FDA had no plans to sample US livestock to see if they carried MRSA.[13]

The FDA may not have performed samples, but Shuaihua Pu and colleagues from Louisiana State University (LSU) did. They took one hundred and twenty raw beef and pork samples randomly from thirty retail grocery stores of seven supermarket chains in Baton Rouge, Louisiana. The results revealed that 40 percent of meats examined contained staphylococcus aureus. Five percent of those contained methicillin-resistant strains.[14]

## MRSA Kills

A study published in the Journal of the American Medical Association estimated that in the year 2005, one hundred thousand MRSA infections occurred in the United States. Of those, nineteen thousand died. That number totals more deaths that year than were caused by HIV/AIDS which was seventeen thousand.[15]Furthermore, MRSA kills more often in the weaker population (children and the elderly), as does *E. coli* 0157:H7.

MRSA should leave us all questioning why it is legal for US farmers to abuse antibiotics that contribute to the growth of resistant strains of bacteria. Estimations made by the Union of Concerned Scientists indicate that 70 percent of antibiotics utilized in the US are for animals, diminishing their efficacy in humans.[16] The FDA estimates the number is larger at 80 percent.[17] The European Union banned the use of antibiotics and related drugs intended for growth promotion purposes on January 1, 2006.[16] How is the country considered the leader of the free world so behind? Unbelievable.

## Fitting It Together

Do you understand the process of how discounting God's design leads to disaster? Is it not amazing how this road to disaster is often paved with greed? Such is the story behind the disasters of *E. coli* 0157:H7 and MRSA. Do you see how eating involves more than just putting convenient foods into our body? Now ask yourself what can I do to protect my family? How can I avoid contributing to these evil practices? The answer is very similar to the previous take-home messages.

**Take-Home Messages and Tips**

**Limit or Eliminate Animal Products**
Avoid meat in your diet, especially ground meat, which is the more common reservoir of *E. coli* 0157:H7. Cook meatless meals for your family. Discuss why you choose to do so with your children.

**Eat Local**

Find local farmers that do not use antibiotics and do use humane rearing and slaughter techniques, if you are going to eat meat.

**Organic**

Organic produce is more expensive. If you have the means, support organic. It will be better for your health. The more that people buy and demand organic produce, the less expensive organic produce will become.

**Grow a Garden**

If you have room, plant a garden. Compost for organic fertilization. (See Appendix C.) Children love planting and working in a garden. They especially love picking the produce.

**Lead**

Teach those around you about the dangers of the meat industry. Help them to protect their own. Protect the weak.

**Pray**

Pray that God would help restore Christ-like values to farming and eating.

# Chapter 6

## Chronic Disease: The Number One Killer of Americans

"There's no question that largely vegetarian diets are as healthy as you can get. The evidence is so strong and overwhelming and produced over such a long period of time that it's no longer debatable."

—Marion Nestle, chair of the nutrition department at New York University

## Number One Chronic Disease

As we discussed, disease can be categorized into two groups; acute and chronic. The next two chapters will discuss two of them more common, most dreaded chronic diseases.

The leading chronic disease contributing to the death of Americans is heart disease. In his book, *The Thrive Diet*, vegan athlete Brendan Brazier puts this into perspective: "According to the American Heart Association, 910,000 Americans die each year due to cardiovascular disease. That's a death-toll equivalent of a 9/11 every 27 hours or a Hurricane Katrina every 17 hours."[1] The most common form of heart disease is coronary artery disease (CAD).[2] In fact, CAD is responsible for more deaths than the top seven leading causes of death combined.[3] How does CAD harm our health?

## Physiology of CAD

Our heart requires oxygen and nutrients supplied from the coronary arteries to live. Healthy arteries have smooth linings with unrestricted blood flow. Many adults' arteries become obstructed through build-up of fat and calcium in the lining. White blood cells try to come to the rescue by adhering to and penetrating the lining in an attempt to ingest the excess fat. The white blood cells then become engorged with bad cholesterol. They eventually form a pus bubble of fat called plaque. These plaques narrow coronary arteries. Blood flows intensely over the plaques causing them to rupture into the blood stream. Because our bodies want to heal the rupture, platelets are sent to clot off the rupture. These clots obstruct flow through the coronary arteries to the heart. If the clot blocks nutrient and oxygen flow to the heart, a portion or all of it will die in a heart attack.[4, 5]

So, if CAD causes heart attack and the greatest loss of life, what causes CAD?

**Cholesterol, Saturated Fat, Trans Fat**

Cholesterol adds to the fat build-up in arteries leading to CAD. Cholesterol in our body basically comes from two sources: our own liver and diet. Humans never need to eat cholesterol since the liver makes it. Cholesterol in our diet always comes from an animal. Check out the levels of cholesterol in these selected foods:

**TABLE 1. Cholesterol Levels in Common Foods**

| Food | Cholesterol (mg) |
|---|---|
| Chicken Breast, cooked (3 oz) | 72 |
| Beef Round, cooked (3 oz) | 71 |
| Pork Chop, cooked (3 oz) | 71 |
| Salmon, baked (3.5 oz) | 87 |
| Egg, whole, large | 212 |
| Cheese Cheddar (3 oz) | 90 |
| Lima Beans | 0 |
| Broccoli | 0 |
| Apple | 0 |

\*\*Source: USDA Nutrient Database and Diet.com.

As demonstrated, the common practice of claiming that "I only eat chicken and fish," does not help regarding cholesterol. Chicken and fish contain cholesterol. Additionally, people love to pull the "genetics" card when it comes to high cholesterol. That is only valid if that person has removed animal products from their diet and made other necessary lifestyle changes such as exercise.

**Saturated Fat**

Saturated fat adds to the fat build-up in arteries leading to CAD. The principal plant sources of saturated fat are coconut oil and coconut milk, palm kernel oil, cocoa butter, and palm oil. From my experience, these are not common cooking oils in the American diet. They can be found in processed foods. The rest of saturated fat comes from an animal. I provide a tip to clients regarding how to know a fat is saturated. It's saturated if it remains solid at room temperature. Think of bacon fat, steak fat, and chicken fat. If you leave them at room temperature, they remain whitish and solid. Another tip? Read the label. It will list saturated fat.

**Trans Fat**

Trans fat adds to the build-up in arteries leading to CAD. It is estimated that a five-gram per day intake of trans fat is associated with a 25 percent increase in the risk of heart disease.[6] Trans fats are not natural; they are made. The process involves adding hydrogen to liquid vegetable oils to make them solid. Food companies use trans fats despite their detriment to our health because they are inexpensive and last. Many fast food restaurants use them to deep-fry foods because they can be used over and over.[7] People need to be aware of trans fats used in fast-food restaurants, and consumers also need to start reading labels. If a label has the phrase "partially hydrogenated oil" listed in the ingredients, the food product contains trans fats.

The above-mentioned fats are items we choose to put into our body. These foods contribute to disease. Not only do they contribute to disease, but also they contribute to heart disease that is killing us. If heart disease does not kill immediately, it can be debilitating. The situation does not have to be this way. Two prominent physicians, Caldwell B. Esselstyn Jr., MD, and Dean Ornish, MD, prove this through their research and patient encounters.

**Caldwell Esselstyn**

The majority of treatment of heart disease occurs after the distressing health event. Chest pains, heart attacks, negative health check-ups lead to stents, bypass surgery, and angioplasty. These have occurred even in my own family. My father went in for a routine life-insurance checkup and received an abnormal electrocardiogram (EKG) test result. Less than two weeks later, he found himself in the hospital recovering from open-heart surgery. He had been diagnosed with high cholesterol levels in the past. He had taken cholesterol-lowering pills. However, he never fixed the underlying problem: he never changed from a diet that diseased his arteries.

Caldwell Esselstyn, Jr., a Cleveland Clinic surgeon and researcher, approaches heart disease differently by tackling the underlying problem. He states, "As a physician, I am embarrassed by my profession's lack of interest in healthier lifestyles. We need to change the way we approach chronic disease." Esselstyn, disenchanted by never curing heart disease or preventing the next casualty, looked for a better way. After scrutinizing epidemiological research, he noticed that in countries where the native diet is low fat and blood-cholesterol levels are below 150 mg/dl (unit of measure for cholesterol: milligrams per deciliter), CAD is rare. Our guidelines in the United States typically recommend blood cholesterol levels to be less than 200. Additionally, autopsies taken of soldiers in the Korean and Vietnam wars revealed the problem with our American diet. Nearly 80 percent of American soldiers had gross evidence of CAD. The arteries of the Asian soldiers were for the most part clean.[5] This reveals two basic realities. One, CAD is not a disease related to age. These were young men. Two, CAD is the result of a poor diet, like the one Americans eat. Because of evidence such as this, Esselstyn tried a different approach.

Esselstyn's treatment guidelines include not eating "anything with a mother or face (no meat, poultry, or fish)." Why? As shown in the above-mentioned information and table 1, they are the source of cholesterol and saturated fat, which are artery-clogging elements. Dairy, oil, and fat are also eliminated. What does he include? He includes vegetables, legumes, whole grains, and fruits. Esselstyn proved through his program, research, and actual angiograms (shown below) that eating this way not only stops CAD but actually reverses it.[5]

## Before    After

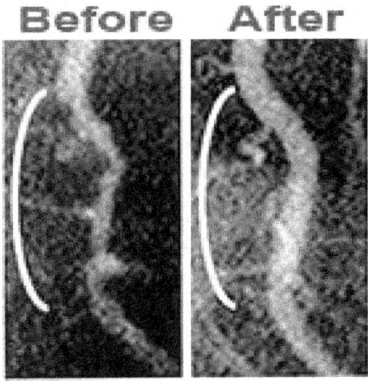

**Source: Caldwell Esselstyn, *Prevent and Reverse Heart Disease*.

The first image was taken November 27, 1996. The second was taken July 22, 1999. Notice how the artery in the second image has opened. This resulted after thirty-two months of a plant-based diet without cholesterol-lowering medication.

Esselstyn's diet plan sounds much like another we have discussed: God's provisions to Adam and Eve. Isn't it amazing how the original diet God gave us in the garden heals us?

## Dean Ornish

Dean Ornish, cardiologist and founder, president and director of the Preventive Medicine Research Institute in Sausalito, California, was at the same time carrying out similar work on the west coast. His program, which also promotes a low-fat (less than 10 percent), vegetarian diet, halts and reverses CAD. He allows fruits, vegetables, grains and legumes with no limitations. Low-fat dairy in moderation is allowed on his plan. Meat and oils are excluded. Again, the plan closely resembles our original God given provision. The plan heals. Ornish's research was so valid, his program so effective, that it became one of the first nonsurgical, nonpharmaceutical plans to be carried by insurance companies.[8]

## Why Haven't You Heard This?

Several reasons exist to clarify why you may have never heard these recommendations: meat and dairy lobbyists, lack of nutrition education in medical schools, and physicians' lack of faith in the public.

**Meat, Dairy, and the USDA**

As I have introduced the USDA in chapter 4, I'll provide governmental guidelines in relation to heart disease. The 2010 USDA guidelines state:

- Consume less than 10 percent of calories from saturated fatty acids by replacing them with monounsaturated and polyunsaturated fatty acids.

- Consume less than 300 mg per day of dietary cholesterol.[9]

When was the last time you calculated the amount of cholesterol you eat on a daily basis? Do you know how many calories are in a gram of fat to enable you to decipher what 10 percent would be? Do you know how to replace saturated fat with poly- or monounsaturated fat? These are supposedly guidelines for the American public.

Considering that all cholesterol and most saturated fat come from animal products, why not just say strictly limit (with easy guidelines) or eliminate animal products from the diet? The answer? The USDA has financial connections to the meat and dairy industry. In fact, the Physicians Committee for Responsible Medicine filed a lawsuit against the USDA for "using deliberately obscure language regarding foods consumers should avoid." They explain, "The Guidelines use biochemical terms, such as 'saturated fat' and 'cholesterol' instead of specific food terms 'meat' and 'cheese.' This deliberate omission can be traced to the USDA's close ties to the meat and dairy industries, including fast-food companies such as McDonald's."[10] This represents one example of many deceptive tactics of the government regarding food.

## Nutrition Education in Medical Schools

American physicians are taught to treat sickness. Prevention of disease is neglected especially with regards to nutrition. A survey of one hundred and six US medical schools was published in the American Journal of Clinical Nutrition. Of these, ninety-nine stated that they required some form of nutrition education. However, only thirty-two required an actual separate course. One course! Only forty of the schools required a minimum of the twenty-five hours of nutrition education recommended by the National Academy of Sciences. Most of the graduating students rated their preparation in nutrition as inadequate. Eighty eight percent of the instructors desired increased nutrition instruction.[11] We definitely need physicians skilled in procedures. However, we also need physicians that prevent the necessity of procedures when possible. At the very least, have skilled dietitians in their offices.

## Physicians Lack of Faith in the Public

Many practitioners do not believe people will change nutrition habits. As a result, many times the truth about nutrition gets watered down. The 2011 American Heart Association guidelines depict this well. The guidelines for cardiovascular disease prevention in women announced a focus on "what works best in the 'real world' vs. clinical research settings."[11] Real-life settings in the United States equate to grabbing high-fat meals at the drive-through. If my mother or sister had gone to a doctor and was given status quo recommendations while the doctor knew the true, effective recommendations, I would be angry to say the least. I cannot practice nutrition that way. As a Christian and a health professional, I am called to tell the truth. That is my responsibility. How my clients respond to that truth is not my responsibility. I can do nothing about that. I love the insight of T. Colin Campbell, one of the authors of *The China Study*:

"If we are reasonably sure of what our data from these studies are telling us, then why must we be reticent about recommending a diet which we know is safe and healthy? Scientists can no longer take the attitude that the public cannot benefit from information they are not ready for. We must have the integrity to tell them the truth and then let them decide. I personally have great faith in the public. We must tell them that a diet of roots, stems, seeds, flowers, fruit, and leaves is the healthiest diet and the only diet we can promote, endorse, and recommend."

I once did a small survey of my dialysis patients. I asked them, "Having been on dialysis and knowing what you know now, what would you have done to prevent this destiny?" Each one said, "Anything!" Then I asked if they would eliminate meat from their diet to prevent it. Each responded with a yes.

God's word is truth. God calls us to be truthful. Valid research done with no financial ties makes us as Campbell states, "reasonably sure." Let these forms of research be your guide. Additionally, look truthfully at your own lifestyle. Is your lifestyle promoting unhealthy arteries? Is the idea of open-heart surgery or a lifetime of medication something you want to avoid? You can.

### Take-Home Messages and Tips

### Limit or Eliminate Animal Products

Animal products are the source of cholesterol and most saturated fat. Limit or eliminate them from your diet.

### Read

Check out books by Caldwell Esselstyn or Dean Ornish. Read information on their websites.

### Seek medical help.

If you currently have high cholesterol or CAD express your desire for aggressive lifestyle therapy. Seek a registered dietitian knowledgeable in plant-based nutrition. Attend one of my classes made affordable online at www.vegwell.com.

### Cook

Get a vegetable-friendly cookbook and brush up on your healthy cooking skills. Cook extra for easy meals to lessen the desire for fast-food.

### Pray

Self-control is a fruit of the spirit. You can pray for it. Pray that God gives you the discipline to eat in a health-promoting way. Pray for friends or family who struggle in this area.

# Chapter 7

## Our Enemy: Cancer

"In a series of experiments, a diet high in animal protein was fed to animals who had been exposed to a cancer-causing toxin. Their liver tumors grew rapidly. However, the tumors stopped growing when animal protein was decreased and replaced with plant proteins. Carcinogenesis – the development of cancer – is turned on by animal protein and turned off by plant protein, even if cancer has already been initiated."

—T. Colin Campbell, PhD

**Declaring War on Cancer**

Cancer is likely the most dreaded of all chronic disease. In 1971, during his State of the Union address, President Nixon declared a war on cancer: "I will also ask for an appropriation of an extra $100 million to launch an intensive campaign to find a cure for cancer, and I will ask later for whatever additional funds can effectively be used. The time has come in America when the same kind of concentrated effort that split the atom and took man to the moon should be turned toward conquering this dread disease. Let us make a total national commitment to achieve this goal."

**Who Is Winning?**

So what is the state of affairs in America regarding cancer today? How far have we come since 1971?

Forty years later, we know more about our enemy. Cancer is not one disease where cells abruptly grow out of control. The American Association for Cancer Research (AACR) reports that cancer more aptly represents two hundred distinct diseases with different causes. Scientists and physicians have improved treatments that extend life for some. However, in 2011 the death rate from cancer is estimated at 571,950 Americans.[1]

With a death toll this high, should we alter the way we fight this war?

**Approaches to War**

In America our initial approach to the war on cancer centers on surveillance and awareness, followed by combat.

Americans refer to mammograms, prostate screenings, colonoscopies, and the like as prevention. What do these procedures do to prevent anything? A more accurate word to describe the procedures is "surveillance." They tell us if the enemy is present.

In the same way, events and walks that raise awareness do not prevent cancer. They help people know the enemy is on the prowl. They raise the flag, and do so effectively. Who does not know what pink ribbons stand for? Awareness has been accomplished well.

I do not have a problem with surveillance or raising awareness. However, these tactics are second steps. The first step is diplomacy. Avoid a war if possible. Neither surveillance nor awareness averts the gruesome combat course of chemotherapy, radiation, amputation, and often death. In order to avoid the war, we need something foreign to our current "sick care" system: prevention.

True prevention halts cancer before it starts. If you examine the main causes of cancer you can see that prevention is possible. Causes of cancer are either hereditary or environmental. Scientists estimate that 75 to 80 percent of cancer stems from environmental causes, meaning we can do something about it! The defeating notion that cancer strikes the unlucky is weakened. We can plan war tactics to keep cancer away from the home front. Of the environmental causes, approximately 2 percent are environmental pollutants, 4 percent are occupational exposures, and 30 percent are from tobacco smoking. The final 35 percent comes from a combination of poor nutrition, physical inactivity, and obesity.[3]

This chapter will focus on preventative measures surrounding nutrition. Scientists estimate that one third of all cancer deaths in America could be prevented through modification of diet.[4] Animal products contribute to cancer growth in our bodies. Fruits and vegetables fight cancer. These two statements help us strategize our prevention plan.

## Meat and Cancer

Many studies reveal a lower incidence of cancer among vegetarians than among meat eaters. Take for example, the study done with The Seventh Day Adventists. The religion encourages a vegetarian diet. However, typically only about 50 percent of the Adventist population avoids meat, so comparisons between two opposing groups are effective. Furthermore, most Adventists do not drink or smoke, eliminating those two factors as confounders to the results. A research series, known as The Adventists Health Studies, investigated diet and the risk of cancer.[5] The research demonstrated overall that avoidance of meat significantly reduces the risk of developing cancer.[6]

Similarly, when reviewing British vegetarians, results indicate total cancer incidence to be lower among vegetarians than meat eaters.[6] Concurrent studies performed in England and Germany demonstrate a 40 percent lower risk of developing cancer in vegetarians over meat eaters.[7, 8, 9, 10]

A study of women in the United Kingdom revealed vegetarian women have a lower risk of breast cancer than meat eaters.[11]

What aspects of meat intake increase the risk of cancer? The answer lies in what meat contains: animal protein, heterocyclic amines (HCA), polycyclic aromatic hydrocarbons (PAH), and nitrates. It also lies in what meat lacks: cancer-protective nutrients.

### Animal Protein—Revelations from The China Study

T. Colin Campbell, Cornell University professor for the division of nutritional sciences, leads the way in cancer research. He was sent to research in the Philippines with a goal of improving childhood nutrition among the poor.

Campbell focused on an unusually high prevalence of liver cancer in these children. All of the children were eating a potent carcinogen from moldy peanuts, aflatoxin. However, to his surprise, the children who ate the most animal protein were the ones getting cancer!

During the course of his research on cancer, Campbell investigated other scientists' data. He noticed a research report from India on rats. In this study, casein, the protein that makes up 87 percent of cow milk protein was given to one set of rats at a rate of 20 percent of their caloric level. They were also given the carcinogen, aflatoxin, the one Filipino children were consuming. The other group was given aflatoxin but the protein level was dropped to 5 percent. Every animal that received the 20 percent protein level got cancer. Every animal that received the 5 percent did not, thus revealing high animal protein intake promotes cancer.

Next, Campbell and colleagues performed a similar study where the rats were given plant-based protein in the form of soy and wheat along with the carcinogen, aflatoxin. This time the protein in both groups was plant based and fed at the rate of 20 percent of caloric intake. Neither group showed early cancer growth, indicating plant-based protein is not cancer promoting.

The grand finale occurred when they fed the rats aflatoxin, as in the India study, and a 20 percent casein diet. All animals fed this diet were dead from liver tumors within one hundred weeks.[12] Campbell's research showed us that in the promotion stage of cancer development, animal protein is potent. His comments? "No chemical carcinogen is nearly so important in causing human cancer as animal protein."

(**I believe in avoiding animal research whenever possible.)

(**It is not possible to feed humans carcinogens, so much of what we calculate evidence from includes animal and epidemiological research.)

## Animal Protein and pH

We have discussed that digestion of animal protein produces an "acid ash," lowering the pH in the body. That acidic environment provides a wonderful breeding ground for cancer cells. Keiichi Morishita, MD, PhD, director of the Ochanomizu Clinic, Japan; head of the International Natural Medicine Association, and author of *The Hidden Truth of Cancer*, states, "If the blood develops a more acidic condition, then these acidic wastes have to be deposited somewhere in the body. It this unhealthy process continues year after year, these areas steadily increase in acidity and their cells begin to die. Other cells in the affected area may survive by becoming abnormal; these are called malignant. Malignant cells cannot respond to brain commands. They undergo a cellular division that is out of control. This is the beginning of cancer." An acidic environment intensifies tumor cell invasion and migration.[13] On the other hand, cancer cells cannot grow in an alkaline environment.[14]

## Heterocyclic Amines (HCA)

As a result of high heat, different foods generate new substances. Many of these are mutagens (a substance or agent that can induce genetic mutation)[15] that cause cancer. One example is HCAs found in cooked meats, chiefly well-done meats. HCAs are extremely powerful mutagens that have induced tumor growth in animal research.

Time and heat determine the amount of HCAs formed in meat. Furthermore, certain HCAs are formed due to high creatine content.[16] All meat has creatine, but not all meat is equal regarding HCA production. See table 1.

**TABLE 1. Five Worst Foods to Grill**

| The 5 Worst Foods to Grill | |
|---|---|
| **Food** | **HCAs ng/100g*** |
| Chicken breast, skinless, boneless, grilled, well done | 14,300 ng/100g[2] |
| Steak, grilled, well done | 810 ng/100g[3] |
| Pork, barbecued | 470 ng/100g[4] |
| Salmon, grilled with skin | 166 ng/100g[5] |
| Hamburger, grilled, well done | 130 ng/100g[3] |
| | |
| *100g portion equals about 3.5 ounces grilled* | |

*Source: Physicians Committee for Responsible Medicine (PCRM), "The 5 Worst Foods to Grill," http://www.pcrm.org/search/?cid=169.

Epidemiological research has mounted over the past ten years regarding carcinogenic meat exposure and cancer risk. A recent review summarizing and evaluating these studies unveil that a high intake of well-done meat containing HCAs may increase the risk of human cancer.[17]

**Polycyclic Aromatic Hydrocarbons (PAH)**

Similar to HCAs, PAHs are formed when cooking meat at high temperatures, particularly grilling. Food for thought: they also come from incomplete burning of coal, oil, gas, and garbage. Think of that when you are ingesting charbroiled meat. When fat from the meat drips onto the hot fire, flames containing PAH flames result. The PAHs cling to the food's exterior. According to the Department of Health and Human Services, PAHs may "reasonably be expected to be carcinogens." A relationship between PAHs and human cancer is widely accepted.[16, 18]

**Nitrates**

I first learned of nitrates as a student at Vanderbilt University Medical Center. We were on a grocery-store tour with our teacher when she raised a package of hot dogs in the air and stated they contained the carcinogen nitrate.

Nitrates are preservatives used in processed meats such as hot dogs to prevent the growth of bacteria. High intake of processed meat containing nitrates is linked to various cancers including those of the colon, the pancreas, and the gastrointestinal tract.[16, 19] Dr. Martin Walker, a leading medical journalist states:

"The truth is processed meats are not a healthful choice for anyone and should be avoided entirely, according to a recent review of more than seven thousand clinical studies examining the connection between diet and cancer. The World Cancer Research Fund (WCRF), using money raised from the general public, commissioned the report. Therefore the findings were not influenced by any vested interests, which makes it all the more reliable. It's the biggest review of the evidence ever undertaken, and it confirms previous findings: Processed meats increase your risk of cancer, especially bowel cancer, and no amount of processed meat is "safe." A previous analysis by the WCRF found that eating just one sausage a day raises your risk of developing bowel cancer by 20%! Other studies have also found that processed meats increase your risk of colon cancer by 50%, bladder cancer by 59%, stomach cancer by 38%, and pancreatic cancer by 67%."

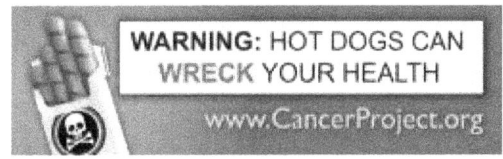

**Source: The Cancer Project.

Animal protein, heterocyclic amines (HCA), polycyclic aromatic hydrocarbons (PAH), and nitrates promote cancer growth. A plan for preventing cancer excludes these items from a person's diet. That is only part of the story. Meat and dairy contain cancer-causing substances, but they are also devoid of cancer-fighting components that are found in plant-based nutrition.

### War Winning Weapon—Plant-Based Nutrition

What do plants have that meat does not have for cancer prevention? They have phytochemicals and antioxidants.

### Phytochemicals

Phytochemicals, nonnutrient compounds found in fruits, vegetables, and grains are biologically active cancer warriors. They act as antioxidants battling free-radical damage in our bodies. What is free-radical damage?

## Free Radicals

All humans on the earth have free radicals in their bodies. They are formed from oxidation. Oxidation results naturally from cellular processes and environmental attacks such as pollution or a poor diet. Free radicals are unstable molecules. They are thieves. Go back to science class, and recall that every molecule has electrons in shells surrounding the nucleus. Free radicals are unhealthy cells missing an electron so they "steal" one from healthy cells.

The once-healthy cell is a free radical. A cascade begins leading to injury of cells. Finally, DNA and tissue are damaged resulting in mutated cancer cells.

Phytochemicals and antioxidants come in as the rescue heroes. They donate an electron to the unstable free radicals, stabilizing them. A great illustration of the process involves an apple. When you cut an apple, it begins to turn brown. That is oxidation. If you were to put lemon juice containing vitamin C, an antioxidant, on the apple, the browning stops. Vitamin C is the rescue hero. Now think of your body. What are you putting in it to stop oxidation? Let's consider some examples of phytochemicals and antioxidants and corresponding food sources.

# TABLE 2. Sources of Phytochemicals and Antioxidants

| Phytochemicals | Examples | Antioxidants Vitamins | Examples |
|---|---|---|---|
| Beta-Carotene | Carrots, Mango | Vitamin A | Broccoli, Sweet Potato |
| Isoflavones | Soy Milk | Vitamin C | Orange, Green Pepper |
| Resveratrol | Red Wine, Purple Grape juice | Vitamin E | Whole Grains, Nuts |
| Lutein | Spinach, Collard Greens | | |
| Lycopene | Tomato Products, Watermelon | | |
| Ellagic Acid | Raspberry, Strawberry | | |

Notice the food sources. While animal products may have trace amounts of some of these nutrients, the prominent sources are plant based.

## Recommendations of Leaders in the War on Cancer

In summary, consider the leading cancer institutions regarding nutrition recommendations for cancer prevention.

American Cancer Society:
- "Limit how much processed meat and red meat you eat."
- "Eat at least 2 1/2 cups of vegetables and fruits each day."[20]

American Institute of Cancer Research:
- "Choose mostly plant foods, limit red meat and avoid processed meat."[21]

World Cancer Research Fund:
- Animal Foods:"Limit intake of red meat and avoid processed meat.
  Public health goal—Population average consumption of red meat to be no more than 300 g (11 oz) a week, very little if any of which is processed.
  Personal recommendation—People who eat red meat to consume less than 500 g (18 oz) a week, very little if any to be processed."
- Plant Foods: "Eat mostly foods of plant origin. Public health goals—Population average consumption of nonstarchy vegetables and of fruits to be at least 600 g (21 oz) daily, relatively unprocessed cereals (grains) and/or pulses (legumes), and other foods that are a natural source of dietary fiber, to contribute to a population average of at least 25 g nonstarch polysaccharide daily."[22]

These recommendations coincide with what I recommend. Again, they are also similar to the original commands of our Lord in the garden and Daniel's diet as we reviewed.

## Take-Home Messages and Tips

### View Cancer Differently

Lose the random-victim mentality. While a healthy lifestyle is not 100 percent protection against cancer, people are also not random victims. What food you choose to put into your body plays a huge role in winning your personal war against cancer.

### Add Nutrition Rescue Heroes

Increase your intake of fruits and vegetables to rescue cells from free-radical damage.

### Avoid Cancer Promoters

Limit or eliminate your intake of animal protein and thus promotion of cancer cells.

### Avoid Carcinogens

Grill less often. When you do grill, try vegetables like portabella mushrooms for example. This will lower your exposure to HCAs and PAHs.

### Eliminate Processed Meat

The research is too strong in this area. I can never recommend eating processed meat. Try veggie dogs, veggie sausage, and tofurkey sandwich meat. These products have great texture and taste.

# Additional Chronic Diseases Considered

Heart disease and cancer may be the most dreaded chronic diseases, but they are not the only ones to consider. We cannot forget conditions such as hypertension (high blood pressure), diabetes, autoimmune disease, and kidney disease. Time and again, research backs up vegetarians and vegans as having lower rates of these diseases. Check out Appendix E for helpful websites regarding a number of the above-mentioned conditions and more.

**Final Thoughts:**

"For the beauty of the earth, for the beauty of the skies…Lord of all to the we raise this our hymn of grateful praise."

My prayer for this book is that eyes will be opened and praise lifted to God and his abundant gifts of this earth. I pray that you realize the considerable bearing our diet has on God's creation. Every meal we eat impacts animals, the environment, and our health—either positively or negatively.

I think of Romans 8:22–25: "We know that the whole creation has been groaning as in the pains of childbirth right up to the present time. Not only so, but we ourselves, who have the first fruits of the Spirit, groan inwardly as we wait eagerly for our adoption to sonship, the redemption of our bodies. For in this hope we were saved. But hope that is seen is no hope at all. Who hopes for what they already have? But if we hope for what we do not yet have, we wait for it patiently."

I can feel the groaning as God's animals are abused in the name of greed, gluttony, and money. I feel loss as our fresh air, water, and land are being destroyed for the same reasons. I have worked with people in agony over their own diseased bodies or those of their loved ones, diseases that could be prevented.

Our current political system is too "crippled to halt nutritional disease epidemics." The officers of the United States Department of Agriculture are prior executives of the cattle, dairy, pork, and egg industries. I do not expect to see aid from the leaders of our country soon if ever.[1]

As Christians we can look to a greater help in times of trouble. Additionally, we have hope for our future. The good news is that Jesus is coming again to restore the earth. His reign will be different.

Revelation 11:15–18 tells us that "the kingdom of the world has become the kingdom of our Lord and of his Messiah, and he will reign for ever and ever. And the twenty-four elders, who were seated on their thrones before God, fell on their faces and worshiped God, saying: "We give thanks to you, Lord God Almighty, the One who is and who was, because you have taken your great power and have begun to reign. The nations were angry, and your wrath has come. The time has come for judging the dead, and for rewarding your servants the prophets and your people who revere your name, both great and small—and for destroying those who destroy the earth."

Isaiah 11:6–9 describes an image of the peaceable kingdom under God's reign:

" The wolf also shall dwell with the lamb, and the leopard shall lie down with the kid; and the calf and the young lion and the fatling together; and a little child shall lead them. And the cow and the bear shall feed; their young ones shall lie down together: and the lion shall eat straw like the ox. And the sucking child shall play on the hole of the asp, and the weaned child shall put his hand on the cockatrice's den. They shall not hurt nor destroy in all my holy mountain: for the earth shall be full of the knowledge of the Lord, as the waters cover the sea."

I long for God's reign and kingdom. Won't you join me in living for his kingdom now? Consider changing your habits. The appendices at the end of this book provide great resources to get started. I teach online classes made affordable for anyone to guide you in your new lifestyle. There are many products available now that make the transition to a plant-based lifestyle easy. I believe in you.

Appeal to your humanity and let's make earth a better place for our children and ourselves, until the Lord's return.

"Thy kingdom come; Thy will be done on earth as it is in heaven."

# Practically Putting It All Together
# Meal Plan and Appendices

**Five Day Meal Plan and Recipes:**
I have learned throughout my years of working with clients that most are not gourmet chefs and have no desire to be. Additionally, people lead busy lives and want quick and easy options. That represents the goal of the below 5 day meal plan. Notice, I have taken the dinner meal from the night before and forwarded it to be the lunch meal of the next day. That saves time. While cleaning up from cooking, go on and make a to-go lunch for the next day. Additionally, most recipes include items that are in most grocery stores. People do not typically want to have to go to several different specialty stores to find products. Many food items can be ordered for home delivery as another option. Descriptions of the meals appear below the meal plan.

**Day 1:**
Breakfast: Coconut Milk Yogurt Parfait, Blueberry Almond Banana Muffin
Lunch: "Chicken" sandwich, Pretzels
Dinner: Black Eye Peas, Southern Yams, Collard Greens, Corn Bread
Snack: Vegan Bar with Peanut Butter, Fruit of Choice
**Day 2:**
Breakfast: Tofu Scramble, Whole Wheat Toast
Lunch: Black Eye Peas, Southern Yams, Collard Greens, Corn Bread
Dinner: Lentil Soup, Strawberry Almond Salad
Snack: Blueberry Almond Banana Muffin, Fruit of Choice
**Day 3:**
Breakfast: Chocolate Covered Strawberry Smoothie
Lunch: Lentil Soup, Strawberry Almond Salad
Dinner: Vegan Fettuccine Alfredo with Gardein Chicken Strips and Mushrooms, Easy Broccoli
Snack: Roasted ChickPeas, Fruit of Choice

**Day 4:**
Breakfast: Vegan Whole Wheat Pancakes
Lunch: Vegan Fettuccine Alfredo with Gardein and Mushrooms, Easy Broccoli
Dinner: Black Beans, Rosemary Asparagus, Easy Yellow Squash,
Snack: Popcorn, Fruit of Choice
**Day 5:**
Breakfast: Cold Cereal with Almond Milk and Blueberries
Lunch: Black Beans, Rosemary Asparagus, Easy Yellow Squash, Field Roast
Dinner: Stuffed Portobello Mushrooms, Baked Potato, Berry Medley
Snack: 1 Handful Almonds (palm of hand) Fruit of Choice

**Coinciding Recipes:**

**Coconut Milk Yogurt Parfait**- Get any flavor coconut milk yogurt (can also use soy) and layer with fruit and granola.

**Blueberry Almond Banana Muffins**-
½ C Smart Balance Light Butter-softened
½ C Agave Nectar
2 Flax Seed Eggs (see below under "further help")
2 Ripe Bananas
1 C All Purpose Flour
1 C Whole Wheat Flour
1 t Baking Soda
½ t salt
1 C Blueberries
Preheat oven to 325. Cream butter and agave nectar. Add "eggs". Beat well. Add next 6 ingredients. Beat well. Fold in blueberries. Bake in either muffin pan or 9x5 loaf pan.

**"Chicken Sandwich"-** Choose any faux chicken meat (Morningstar farms, Gardein) Prepare the same way you would if you were using meat. Make a sandwich using a whole wheat bun. Get creative! Add avacados, fresh oregano, vegan cheese, etc…

**Black Eye Peas and Collard Greens**-I love a product called "Not Chick'n" by Edward and Sons. I have found it at most local grocery stores. I only use ¼ a cube to lower the sodium content. It makes all vegetables like peas and greens amazing. No more adding fatty bacon or ham.

**Southern Yams-** Peel and slice the number of yams you desire. Melt Smart Balance Light spread in a large skillet. Add the yams. Drizzle Agave Nectar over the top for desired level of sweetness. Then cook until the yams are soft and brown. Depending on the amount you cook it typically takes around 30 minutes. Agave nectar can be found at most local grocery stores near the sugar and sweeteners. It is lower in calories and natural. It is similar in appearance to pancake syrup or honey.

**Vegan Corn Bread-**
¾ C Yellow Cornmeal
½ C Oat Bran
1/3 C Whole Wheat Flour
2 t Baking Powder
½ t Salt
¼ t Baking Soda
1 T Agave Nectar
1 C Almond Milk-Plain
¼ C Unsweetened Applesauce

Preheat oven to 425 degrees F. Mix together the cornmeal, oat bran, whole wheat flour, baking powder salt, baking soda in a medium sized bowl.
Add the agave nectar, almond milk, and applesauce. Stir until mixed. Use nonstick spray to coat an 8" x 8" pan. Pour batter into pan and bake for 15 minutes until golden.

**Vegan Bar-** When choosing a health bar, be sure it is actually healthy. Watch for animal ingredients such as whey, casein, milk, etc… Also ensure there are no partially hydrogenated oils of any kind.

**Tofu Scramble-** Scrambled tofu is used as a replacement for scrambled eggs by many. There are hundreds of recipes with different spices. Look up several on the internet and choose the one spiced to your taste.

**Lentil Soup-**
1 C Lentils
2 C Vegetable Broth
3 C Water
1 Onion, chopped
1 C Tomato Sauce
1 T Minced Garlic
1 t Pepper
1 Celery Stalk Chopped
2 Carrots Chopped
¼ t Oregano
Put lentils in pot with vegetable broth and water. Bring to a boil. Add all other ingredients. Reduce heat. Cover and simmer for 1 ½ hours.

**Strawberry Almond Salad-** Simply choose a type of lettuce. I love spring mix. Slice fresh strawberries and purple onion on top. Add a handful of almonds. For a dressing I love a tablespoon of olive oil, red wine vinegar (around ¼ cup depending on the salad size), minced garlic, and dried oregano. Just mix the ingredient together and pour over the salad.

**Chocolate Covered Strawberry Smoothie-** Put around a cup of frozen strawberries in a blender along with a vegan protein powder of choice (I prefer rice or a blend. Soy causes gastrointestinal upset for many). Add 1 tablespoon of cocoa powder, and vegan milk to desired level of consistency. I usually add around 1 cup as I like it thick. Blend together and enjoy.

**Vegan Fettuccine Alfredo-**
8 ounces fettuccine (use less if you like it extra saucy)
5 tablespoons Smart Balance Light Butter
1/2 package (4 ounces) vegan cream
1 cup unsweetened nondairy milk (I use almond milk)
3 1/2 tablespoons vegan parmesan cheese
   1 1/2 teaspoons garlic powder
   1/2 teaspoon ground white or black pepper
   1/2 cup vegan mozzarella
   salt and pepper to taste

Cook pasta according to package directions.Melt the butter in a saucepan over medium heat. Add the cream cheese and whisk until smooth. Whisk in the milk gradually. Mix in the parmesan, garlic powder, salt, pepper. Add the mozzarella and continue to stir until it's completely melted.
Pour over pasta and combine.

**Easy Broccoli-** Put desired amount of broccoli **florets** in a glass bowl. Add water to the half way mark. Add several pats of Smart Balance Light butter to the top with a sprinkle of salt. Microwave for 5 minutes 30 seconds or until heated.

**Roasted Chick Peas-** Preheat oven to 400. Open and drain desired number of cans of chick peas. Pour the peas into a plastic bag and sprinkle generously with your favorite seasoning. Being from the Memphis Area, I love Rendezvous Dry Barbeque Rub. Spread the peas out flat on a cookie sheet. Cook until crunchy.

**Vegan Whole Wheat Pancakes-**

1 C Whole Wheat Flour

1 C All Purpose Flour

1 ½ T Baking Powder

½ t Salt

2 T Agave Nectar

2 Flax Seed Eggs (see "Further Help" below)

2 C Almond Milk

1 T Canola Oil

In a Large bowl stir together first 4 dry ingredients. In another bowl mix remaining wet ingredients. Add the wet to the dry. Stir until blended.  Pour about ½ C of batter onto a skillet or griddle lightly sprayed with nonstick spray. Cook over medium heat until golden.

**Black Beans-** Heat a teaspoon of olive oil and a tablespoon of minced garlic in a saucepan until aromatic. Add ½ chopped onion or ½ cup frozen chopped onion, diced tomatoes (canned or fresh), and black beans (1 can or 2 cups). Heat for 20 minutes.

**Rosemary Asparagus-** Remove hard tips from asparagus and lay out flat on a cookie sheet. Sprinkle with olive oil. Lay fresh rosemary across the top and sprinkle with salt and pepper. Heat at 400 for 20-30 minutes or desired consistency.

**Easy Squash-** Slice yellow squash in ¼- ½ inch thick circles. Place squash in a skillet with 2 tablespoons Smart Balance Light spread. Sprinkle small amount of season salt or Mrs Dash. Cook for 20-30 minutes or desired consistency.

**Stuffed Portobello Mushrooms-** Mix ½ cup vegan cream cheese (Tofutti is great. This can be found at whole foods. If you do not have access to Whole foods just season the mushroom) with 1 diced green onion, 1 tablespoon minced garlic. Brush the mushroom with Worcestershire or light soy sauce. Fill with cream cheese mixture. Slice large tomato and place on top. Place mushrooms in a skillet (preferable cast iron). Sauté in olive oil for 10 minutes then place the entire skillet in oven at 400 for 20 more minutes.

## Further Help: Veggie Substitutions for Your Favorite Recipes

**For Cheese or Cream Cheese Try**: Brands include Daiya, Galaxy, Vegan Gourmet, Follow Your Heart
**For Milk Try:** Almond Milk, Coconut Milk, Soy Milk, Rice Milk-numerous brands
**For Chicken Try:** Brands include Gardein, Morningstar Farms, Boca
**For Ground Beef Try:** Brands include Smart Grounds and Gimme Lean by Lightlife, Yves, Morningstar Farms, Boca
**For Eggs Try:** Ener G egg replacer which is better for desserts.  Make a homemade egg: 1 tablespoon of ground flaxseed to 3 tablespoons water. This works great in whole wheat recipes such as pancakes.

Taken from Climbing For Christ. Find out more about their ministry at: http://www.climbingforchrist.org/

## Four Biblical Principles for Environmental Stewardship By Calvin B. DeWitt

1. Earth keeping Principle

AS THE LORD KEEPS AND SUSTAINS US, SO MUST WE KEEP AND SUSTAIN OUR LORD'S CREATION.

Genesis 2:15 expects Adam and Adam's descendants to serve and keep the garden. The Hebrew word upon which the translation of keep is based is the word "shamar" and "shamar" means a loving, caring, sustaining keeping. This word also is used in the Aaronic blessing, from Numbers 6:24, "The Lord bless you and keep you." When we invoke God's blessing to keep us, it is not merely that God would keep us in a kind of preserved, inactive, uninteresting state. Instead, it is that God would keep us in all of our vitality, with all our energy and beauty. The keeping we expect of God when we invoke the Aaronic blessing is one that nurtures all of our life-staining and life-fulfilling relationships — with our family, spouse, and children, with our neighbors and our friends, with the land and creatures that sustain us, with the air and water, and with our God.

And so too with our keeping of the Garden — in our keeping of God's Creation. When Adam, Eve, and we, keep the Creation, we make sure that the creatures under our care and keeping are maintained with all their proper connections — connections with members of the same species, with the many other species with which they interact, with the soil, air and water upon which they depend. The rich and full keeping that we invoke with the Aaronic blessing is the kind of rich and full keeping that we should bring to the garden of God — to God's creatures and to all of Creation. As God keeps believing people, so should God's people keep Creation.

2. Sabbath Principle

WE MUST PROVIDE FOR CREATION'S SABBATH RESTS.

Exodus 20 and Deuteronomy 5 require that one day in seven be set aside as a day of rest for people and for animals. As human beings and animals are to be given their times of sabbath rest, so also is the land. Exodus 23 commands, "For six years you shall sow your land and gather in its yield; but the seventh year you shall let it rest and lie fallow, that the poor of your people may eat; and what they leave the wild beasts may eat." "You may ask, 'What will we eat in the seventh year if we do not plant or harvest our crops?'" God's answer in Leviticus 25 and 26 is: "I will send you such a blessing in the sixth year that the land will yield enough for three years," so do not worry, but practice this law so that your land will be fruitful. "If you follow my decrees and are careful to obey my commands, I will send you rain in its season, and the ground will yield its crops and the trees of the field their fruit."

Christ in the New Testament clearly teaches that the Sabbath is made for the ones served by it — not the other way around. Thus, the sabbath year is given to protect the land from relentless exploitation, to help the land rejuvenate, to help it get things together again; it is a time of rest and restoration. This sabbath is not merely a legalistic requirement; rather, it is a profound principle. Thus in some Christian farming communities, the sabbath principle is practiced by letting the land rest every second year, "because that is what the land needs." And of course, it is not therefore restricted to agriculture but applies to all Creation. The Bible warns in Leviticus 26, "...if you will not listen to me and carry out all these commands, and if you reject my decrees and abhor my laws and fail to carry out all my commands and so violate my covenant, ...Your land will be laid waste, and your cities will lie in ruins... Then the land will enjoy its sabbath years all the time it lies desolate... then the land will rest and enjoy its sabbaths. All the time that it lies desolate, the land will have the rest it did not have during the sabbaths you lived in it."

3. Fruitfulness Principle

WE SHOULD ENJOY, BUT MUST NOT DESTROY, CREATION'S FRUITFULNESS.

The fish of the sea and the birds of the air, as well as people, are given God's blessing of fruitfulness. In Genesis 1:20 and 22 God declares, "Let the water teem with living creatures, and let birds fly above the earth across the expanse of the sky." And then God blesses these creatures with fruitfulness: "Be fruitful and increase in number and fill the water in the seas, and let the birds increase on the earth." God's Creation reflects God's fruitful work — God's fruitful work of giving what satisfies to the land and waters and their abundant life. As it is written in Psalm 104, "He makes springs pour water into the ravines; it flows between the mountains. They give water to all the beasts of the field; the wild donkeys quench their thirst. The birds of the air nest by the waters; they sing among its branches. He waters the mountains from his upper chambers; the earth is satisfied by the fruit of his work." And Psalm 23 describes how our providing God "... makes me lie down in green pastures, ... leads me beside quiet waters, ... restores my soul."

As God's fruitful work brings fruit to Creation, so too should ours. As God provides for the creatures, so should we people who were created to reflect God whose image we bear. Imaging God, we too should provide for the creatures. And, as Noah spared no time, expense, or reputation when God's creatures were threatened with extinction, neither should we. Deluges — in Noah's time of water, and in our time of floods of people and environmental degradation — sprawl over the land, displacing God's creatures, limiting their potential to obey God's command, "be fruitful and increase in number." To those who would allow this to happen, the prophet Isaiah warns: "Woe to you who add house to house and join field to field till no space is left and you live alone in the land" (Isaiah 5:8).

Thus, while expected to enjoy Creation, while expected to partake of Creation's fruit, we may not destroy the fruitfulness upon which Creation's fullness depends. We must, with Noah, save and keep the species whose interactions with each other, and with land and water, form the fabric of the biosphere. We should let the profound admonition of Ezekiel 34:18 reverberate and echo in our minds:

"Is it not enough for you to feed on the green pastures? Must you also trample them with your feet? "Is it not enough for you to drink the pure water? Must you also muddy it with your feet?"

4. Con-Servancy Principle

WE MUST RETURN CREATION'S SERVICE TO US WITH SERVICE OF OUR OWN.

This principle overarches all the others. The word *conservancy* refers to conservation and often denotes an organization that regulates fisheries and/or protects other natural resources. We can hyphenate this word to draw attention to its root meaning—*con* + *serve*—meaning "to serve with."

From earthkeeping principle, we noted from Genesis 2:15 that Adam and Adam's descendants were expected to be "guardeners," responsible gardeners commissioned to *serve* the garden and to *keep* it. The Hebrew word *'abad* ("serve") in this passage occurs 290 times in the Old Testament, and it is most often translated as "serve," as in Joshua 24:15: "Choose for yourselves this day whom you will serve. . . . As for me and my household, we will serve the LORD."

The various Bible translations of *'abad* in Genesis 2:15—"serve," "till," "dress," and "work"—relate to worthy service. God calls us to give the garden of creation our caring service.

We already know from experience with the "beautiful book" of creation that this garden serves us. It serves us with good food, beauty, herbs, fiber, medicine, pleasant microclimates, continual soil-making, nutrient processing, and seed production. The garden and the larger biosphere provide what ecologists call "ecosystem services" such as water purification by evaporation and percolation, moderation of flood peaks and drought flows by river-system wetlands, development of soils from the weathering of rocks, sequestration of excess atmospheric carbon dioxide in wetland peats and fossil carbon, and moderation of local climates by nearby bodies of water. Yet Genesis addresses *our* service to the garden. The garden's service *to us* is implicit; service *from us* to the garden is explicit.

Like Adam and Adam's descendants, we are expected to return the service of the garden with service of our own. This is a reciprocal service, a "service with"—in other words, a *con-service*, a *con-servancy*, a *con-servation*. This reciprocal service defines an engaging relationship between garden and gardener, between the biosphere and its safeguarding stewards.

So we can call this "never taking from creation without returning service of our own" the *Con-Servancy Principle* (or *Con-Servation Principle*). Our love of our Creator God, God's love of the creation, and our imaging this love of God—all join together to commission us as *con-servers* of creation. As *con-servers*, we follow the example of the final Adam—Jesus Christ (see 1 Cor. 15:22, 45) by whom God created, sustains, and reconciles all things (see Col. 1:15-20).

Calvin B. DeWitt is Professor of Environmental Studies at the University of Wisconsin-Madison and is past Director and President of Au Sable Institute of Environmental Studies which serves 60 Christian colleges and universities with courses and programs in environmental stewardship in Michigan, Puget Sound, Costa Rica, and India. Dr. DeWitt has been a Charles H. Spurgeon Guest Lecturer at Denver Seminary, Francis Schaeffer Lecturer at Covenant Seminary, and Abraham Kuyper Lecturer at Fuller Theological Seminary.

Dr. DeWitt is a member of the Teaching Academy and received the Chancellor's Award for Distinguished Teaching at the University of Wisconsin where he is a member of the graduate faculties of Environment and Resources, Water Resources Management, Limnology and Marine Science, and Conservation Biology and Sustainable Development. His technical publications are in environmental physiology, wetlands ecology, environmental stewardship, and biblical environmental teachings. His current work is focused on the integration of science and environmental ethics in application to practice and ecological sustainability. His books include Missionary Earthkeeping (Mercer University Press, 1992, with Ghillean T. Prance), Caring for Creation (Baker Books, 1997), Earthwise: A Hopeful Guide to Creation Care, $3^{rd}$ edition, 2011 (Faith Alive Christian Resources, 2011), and Song of A Scientist Square Inch Books, 2012.

**Appendix B:**

**Steps to Recycling a Product**

Recycling includes collecting recyclable materials that would otherwise be considered waste, sorting and processing recyclables into raw materials such as fibers, manufacturing raw materials into new products, and purchasing recycled products.

Collecting and processing secondary materials, manufacturing recycled-content products, and then buying recycled products creates a circle or loop that ensures the overall success and value of recycling.

### *Step 1. Collection and Processing*
Collecting recyclables varies from community to community, but there are four primary methods: curbside, drop-off centers, buy-back centers, and deposit/refund programs.

Regardless of the method used to collect the recyclables, the next leg of their journey is usually the same. Recyclables are sent to a materials recovery facility to be sorted and prepared into marketable commodities for manufacturing. Recyclables are bought and sold just like any other commodity, and prices for the materials change and fluctuate with the market.

### Step 2. Manufacturing

Once cleaned and separated, the recyclables are ready to undergo the second part of the recycling loop. More and more of today's products are being manufactured with total or partial recycled content. Common household items that contain recycled materials include newspapers and paper towels; aluminum, plastic, and glass soft drink containers; steel cans; and plastic laundry detergent bottles. Recycled materials also are used in innovative applications such as recovered glass in roadway asphalt (glassphalt) or recovered plastic in carpeting, park benches, and pedestrian bridges.

### Step 3. Purchasing Recycled Products

Purchasing recycled products completes the recycling loop. By "buying recycled," governments, as well as businesses and individual consumers, each play an important role in making the recycling process a success. As consumers demand more environmentally sound products, manufacturers will continue to meet that demand by producing high-quality recycled products. Learn more about recycling terminology and to find tips on identifying recycled products.

**Appendix C:**
**Composting**
**What to Compost – The IN List**
Animal manure
Cardboard rolls
Clean paper
Coffee grounds and filters
Cotton rags
Dryer and vacuum cleaner lint
Eggshells
Fireplace ashes
Fruits and vegetables
Grass clippings
Hair and fur
Hay and straw
Houseplants
Leaves
Nut shells
Sawdust
Shredded newspaper
Tea bags
Wood chips
Wool rags
Yard trimmings

**What Not to Compost – The OUT List**
**Leave Out/Reason Why**
Black walnut tree leaves or twigs:
Releases substances that might be harmful to plants
Coal or charcoal ash:
 Might contain substances harmful to plants
Dairy products (e.g., butter, milk, sour cream, yogurt) and eggs: Create odor problems and attract pests such as rodents and flies
Diseased or insect-ridden plants: Diseases or insects might survive and be transferred back to other plants
Fats, grease, lard, or oils: Create odor problems and attract pests such as rodents and flies
Meat or fish bones and scraps: Create odor problems and attract pests such as rodents and flies
Pet wastes (e.g., dog or cat feces, soiled cat litter): Might contain parasites, bacteria, germs, pathogens, and viruses harmful to humans
Yard trimmings treated with chemical pesticides: Might kill beneficial composting organisms
**\*\*Composting.EPA Website.**

**Resources Appendix B and C:**

http://www.benefits-of-recycling.com/definitionofcomposting.html
http://www.epa.gov/osw/conserve/rrr/composting/index.htm
http://www.epa.gov/osw/conserve/rrr/composting/questions.htm
http://www.epa.gov/osw/conserve/rrr/composting/benefits.htm

**Appendix D**:
**Resources for feeding children:**

Feeding Vegan Kids by Reed Mangels, Ph.D., R.D. available at:
http://www.vrg.org/nutshell/kids.htm

A Weekly Menu Plan for Vegetarian Kid Friendly Meals available
at: http://www.savvyvegetarian.com/blog/advice/a-week-of-
menus-for-vegetarian-kid-friendly-meals

Book-New Vegetarian Baby by Sharon A. Yntema and Christine
Beard

Book-Raising Vegetarian Children by Joanne Stepaniak, MS
ED and Vesanto Melina, MS, RD.

## Veg Friendly Meat and Dairy Alternatives for kids:

"Chicken Nuggets": brands include Morningstar Farms, Gardein,
Boca, Trader Joes

"Sandwich Meat": Brands include Tofurkey, Lightlife Smart Deli

"Cheese": Brands include Daiya, Galaxy, Vegan Gourmet, Follow
Your Heart

"Butter": Smart Balance Light (the regular is not vegan), Earth
Balance

"Milk": Almond Milk, Coconut Milk, Soy Milk, Rice Milk-
numerous brands

"Yogurt": Brands include So Delicious, Silk, Wholesoy,

**Appendix E:**
**Helpful Websites:**

T.Collin Campbell Foundation-www.tcolincampbell.org

Dr. McDougall's Health and Medical Center-
http://www.drmcdougall.com

Preventative Medicine Research Institute-
http://www.pmri.org/dean_ornish.html

Prevent and Reverse Heart Disease-
http://www.heartattackproof.com

The Cancer Project-http://www.cancerproject.org/

PCRM: Physicians Committee for Responsible Medicine-
http://www.pcrm.org/

John Robbins Official Site- http://www.johnrobbins.info/

Jenn E Moore official website-http://www.Vegwell.com

The Vegetarian Resource Group- http://www.vrg.org

Vegan Health Home Page-http://www.veganhealth.org/

A Well Fed World- http://www.awellfedworld.org/

Johns Hopkins Center for a Livable Future-
http://www.jhsph.edu/clf/

Mercy For Animals-http://www.mercyforanimals.org/

Farm Animal Rights Movement-
http://www.greenyourdiet.org

**References:**

Chapter 1

1. Lappe' A. The Climate Crises at the End of Our Fork. In: Weber K. ed. *Food INC.* New York, NY: PublicAffairs; 2009:110.
2. Robbins J. *Diet For a New America.* Walpole, NH: Stillpoint Publishing; 1987.
3. Animals Unleashed web site. Available at: http://www.unleashed.org.au/animals/pigs.php. Accessed October 10, 2011.
4. VIVA! USA Pig Appeal website. Available at: http://www.vivausa.org/campaigns/pigs/report.htm. Accessed October 20, 2011.
5. Hudson WH. *The Book of a Naturalist.* New York, NY: George H Duran Co. 1919.
6. Brynes J. Raising Pigs By The Calendar At Maplewood Farm. *Hog Farm Management*. September 1976;30.
7. Robbins J. *Food Revolution*. Berkeley, CA: Conari Press. 2001.
8. Global Action Network-Cows web site. Available at: http://www.gan.ca/animals/cows.en.html. Accessed October 05, 2011.
9. Vegan Outreach. Why Vegan-Boycott Cruelty. Vegan Outreach Brochure. 2009.
10. The Pain of Debeaking-Free Range Farmers Inc web site. Available at: http://www.freerangefarmers.com.au/debeaking.htm. November 1, 2011.
11. Continuing Problems in USDA's enforcement of the Humane Methods of Slaughter Act. Statement of Wayne Pacelle President and CEO-The Humane Society of the United States to Domestic Policy Subcommittee. 2009.

12. Continuing Problems in USDA's enforcement of the Humane Methods of Slaughter Act. Statement of Dean Wyatt FSIS Supervisory Public Health Veterinarian to Domestic Policy Subcommittee. 2010.
13. United States Code Website. Chapter 48 Humane Methods of Livestock Slaughter. Available at: http://uscode.house.gov/download/pls/07C48.txt. Accessed June 6, 2011.

Chapter 2

1. Carlsson-Kanyama A, Gonzalez AD. Potential contributions of food consumption patterns to climate change. *Am J Clin Nutr.* 2009;89(suppl):1704s-9s.
2. Taskforce Report. *Preparing U.S. Agriculture for Global Climate Change.* 1992. No.119. Ames, IA: Council for Agricultural Science and Technology
3. National Council for Agricultural Education. *Global Climate Change and Environmental Stewardship by Ruminant Livestock Producers:* 1998. Agricultural Education University of Missouri.
4. Dictionary.com website. *The American Heritage® Science Dictionary*. Houghton Mifflin Company. Available at: http://dictionary.reference.com/browse/greenhouse effect . Accessed August 24, 2011.
5. Lomborg B. *Cool It-The Skeptical Environmentalists Guide to Global Warming.* New York, NY: Random House Inc. 2008.

6.  Braasch G, McKibben B. *Earth Under Fire: How Global Warming is Changing the World*. Berkeley, CA: University of California Press. 2009.

7.  Cool Foods Campaign. Another Take, Global Warming and Your Food. In: Weber K ed. Food INC. New York, NY: Public Affairs; 2009:121.

8.  Bittman M. *Food Matters*. New York, NY: Simon and Schuster. 2009.

9.  International Carbon Bank and Exchange web site. Calculating Greenhouse Gases. Available at: http://www.icbe.com/emissions/calculate.asp. Accessed on September 2, 2011.

10. Koneswaran G, Nierenberg D. Commentary: Global Farm Animal Production and Global Warming: Impacting and Mitigating Climate Change. *Environ Health Perspect.* 2008;116:578-582.

11. National Pollutant Discharge Elimination System permit regulation and effluent limitation guidelines and standards for concentrated animal feeding operations (CAFOs);final rule. Fed Reg 68:7175-7274.

12. Paustian K, Antle M, Sheehan J, Eldor P. Pew Center on Global Climate Change. *Agriculture's Role in Greenhouse Gas Emission*. Washington DC;2006.

13. Steinfeld H, Gerber P, Wassenaar T, Castel V, Rosales M, de Haan C. Food and Agriculture Organization of the United Nations. *Livestock's Long Shadow: environmental issues and options*. Rome, Italy; 2006.

14. The Environmental Beef With Meat. *The Bay Weekly*. January 6, 2005.
15. Smithsonian Institution. Smithsonian Researchers Show Amazonian Deforestation Accelerating. *Science Daily* [online]. January 15, 2002.
16. Mongabay web site. Global Consequences of Deforestation in the Tropics. Available at: http://rainforests.mongabay.com/0901.htm. Accessed on July 8, 2011.
17. Children's Tropical Forests web site. Children's Tropical Forests (UK) Factsheet. Available at: http://ds.dial.pipex.com/ctf/facts/plants.htm. Accessed on July 8, 2011.
18. Rain-tree website. Rainforest Facts. Available at: http://www.rain-tree.com/facts.htm. Accessed on July 8, 2011.
19. Food and Agricultural Association Paper Reports. Turner K, Georgio S, Clark R, Brower R, Burke J. *Economic valuation of water resources in agriculture, From the Sectoral to a functional perspective of natural resource management*. 2004. No. 27. FAO. Rome;2004.
20. Gerber P, Menzi H. Nitrogen Losses from intensive livestock farming systems in Southeast Asia: A Review of current trends and mitigation options. *International Congress Series* (online). 2005;1293:253-261. Available from: Science Direct. Accessed September 12, 2011.
21. Stathopoulos AS. You Are What Your Food Eats: How Regulation of Factory Farm Conditions Could Improve Human Health and Animal Welfare Alike. *13 N.Y.U. J. Legis. 7 Pub. Pol'y 407*, 2010. Available

at Gibbons Law web site. Accessed on August 12, 2011.

22. University of Nevada Cooperative Extension web site. Liquid Manure Storage Treatment Options, Including Lagoons. Available at: http://www.extension.org/pages/19941/liquid-manure-storage-treatment-options. Accessed on August 12, 2011.

23. Natural Resources Defense Council web site. Pollution from Giant Livestock Farms Threatens Public Health. Available at: http://www.nrdc.org/water/pollution/nspills.asp. Accessed on July 30, 2011.

24. Wisconsin Stewardship Network web site. Fact Sheet: The Environmental Impact of Factory Farms. Available at: http://www.wsn.org/factoryfarm/factfarmfactsheet.html. Accessed on July 30, 2011.

Chapter 3

1. VegSource web site. The Comparative Anatomy of Eating.  Available at: Http://www.vegsource.com/news/2009/11/the-comparative-anatomy-of-eating.html. Accessed on September 20, 2011.

2. Winnipeg Assembly of Yahweh web site. Carnivores vs Herbivores.  Ten Physical Differences Between Carnivores (MeatEaters) and Herbivores (Plant Eaters).  Is the Human Body Designed To Eat Animal Products? Available at: http://www.waoy.org/26.html. Accessed on September 20, 2011.

1. Race and History web site. Got Milk White Poison. Available at: http://www.raceandhistory.com/cgi-bin/forum/webbbs_config.pl/noframes/read/14. Accessed on October 10, 2011.
2. USDA web site. Dietary Guidance. Available at: http://fnic.nal.usda.gov/nal_display/index.php?info_center=4&tax_level=3&tax_subject=256&topic_id=1348&level3_id=5715. Accessed on October 10, 2010.
3. Food and Nutrition Service (FNS), U.S. Department of Agriculture web site. *Average Percentage for School Purchase Planning and Ordering*. Powerpoint Slide. Alexandria, VA: FNS; 2008.
4. Opensecrets web site. Top Contributors. Available at: http://www.opensecrets.org/index.php. Accessed on October 24, 2011.
5. PCRM Website. Agriculture and Health Policies in Conflict-How Ag subsidies Tax Our Health. Available at: http://www.pcrm.org/health/reports/agriculture-and-health-policies-conclusion. Accessed on October 24, 2011.
6. USDA web site. Special Milk Program. Available at: http://www.fns.usda.gov/cnd/milk/. Accessed on October 24, 2011.
7. Milk ProCon web site. Should milk be a part of a federally subsidized school program. Available at: http://milk.procon.org/view.answers.php?questionID=000841. Accessed on October 27, 2011.
8. Heyman MB. Lactose Intolerance in Infants, Children, and Adolescents. *Pediatrics*. September 2006;118(3):1279-1286.
9. Lanou AJ. Should dairy be recommended as part of a healthy vegetarian diet? *Am J Clin Nutr*. 2009;89(suppl):1638S-42S.

10. National Institutes of Health web site. News Release NIH. "Calcium Crises' affects American Youth: Extended Web site seeks to inform children of the dangers of low calcium intake. Available at: http://www.nih.gov/news/pr/dec2001/nichd-10.htm. Accessed November 1, 2011.

11. Dr. Mark Hyman web site. Dairy: 6 Reasons You Should Avoid It at all Costs. Available at: http://drhyman.com/dairy-6-reasons-you-should-avoid-it-at-all-costs-2943/. Accessed on on October 25, 2011.

12. Speaking Out against Dairy website. Available at: http://www.stott.net/articles/show/210217-Speaking-out-against-Dairy. Accessed on November 6, 2011.

13. Lanou AJ, Berkow SE, Barnard ND. Calcium, Dairy Products, and Bone Health in Children and Young Adults: A Reevaluation of the Evidence. *Pediatrics.* 2005;115(3):736-743.

14. Lloyd T, Chinchilli VM, Johnson-Rollings N, Kieselhorst K, Eggli DF, Marcus R. Adult Female Hip Bone Density Reflects Teenage Sports-Exercise Patterns But Not Teenage Calcium Intake. *Pediatrics.* 2000;106(1): 40-44.

15. Spock B. *Dr. Spock's Baby and Child Care. 9th ed.* New York, NY. Gallery Books; 2011.

16. Lloyd T, Chinchilli VM, Johnson-Rollings N, Kieselhorst K, Eggli DF, Marcus R. Adult Female Hip Bone Density Reflects Teenage Sports-Exercise Patterns But Not Teenage Calcium Intake. *Pediatrics.* 2000;106(1): 40-44.

17. Drash AL, Kramer MS, Swanson J, Udall JN. American Academy of Pediatrics Infant Feeding Practices and Their Possible Relationship to the Etiology of Diabetes Mellitus. *Pediatrics.* 1994;94(5):752-754.

18. Gerstein HC. Cow's milk exposure type 1 diabetes mellitus. A critical overview of the clinical literature. *Diabetes Care.* 1994;17:13-19.
19. Schrezenmeir J, Jagla A. Milk and Diabetes. *J Am Col of Nutr.* 2000;19(suppl)(2): 176(S)-190(S).
20. Harvard School of Public Health web site.The Nutrition Source Food Pyramids and Plates: What Should You Really Eat? Harvard School of Public Health. Available at: http://www.hsph.harvard.edu/nutritionsource/what-should-you-eat/pyramid-full-story/index.html. Accessed on November 5, 2011.
21. Feskanich D, Willett WC, Stampfer MJ, Colditz GA. Milk, Dietary Calcium, and Bone Fractures in Women: A 12-Year Prospective Study. *Am J Public Health.* 1997;87(6): 992-997.
22. Sellmeyer D, Stone KL, Sebastian A, Cummings SR. A high ratio of dietary animal to vegetable protein increases the rate of bone loss and the risk of fracture in postmenopausal women. *Am J Clin Nutr.* January 2001;73(1):118-122.
23. USDA website. USDA DRI Tables. Available at: http://fnic.nal.usda.gov/nal_display/index.php?info_center=4&tax_level=3&tax_subject=256&topic_id=1342&level3_id=5140. Accessed on November 5, 2011.

Chapter 5

1. Brazier B. *Thrive Fitness*. Canada: The Penguin Group. 2009.
2. Centers for Disease Control and Prevention web site. Heart Disease Facts. Available at: http://www.cdc.gov/heartdisease/facts.htm. Accessed on January 4, 2012.
3. Singh VN. Coronary Artery Disease Overview. *EMedicine Health*(online). Available at:

144

http://www.emedicinehealth.com/coronary_hear t_disease_/article_em.htm. Accessed on January 4, 2012.

4.  Mayo Clinic web site. Heart Attack. Available at: http:/www.mayoclinic.com/health/heart-attack/DS00094/METHOD=print. Accessed on January 4, 2012.

5.  Esselstyn C Jr. *Prevent and Reverse Heart Disease*. New York, NY: Penguin Group; 2008.

6.  Stender S, Dyerberg J. High Levels of Industrial Produced Trans Fat in Popular Fast Foods. *New Eng J of Med*. 2006;354:15.

7.  American Heart Association web site. TransFats. Available at: http://www.heart.org/HEARTORG/GettingHealthy /FatsAndOils/Fats101/Trans-Fats_UCM_3-112-_Article.jsp. Accesses 1/5/2012. Accessed on January 7, 2012.

8.  **http://www.ornishspectrum.com/.** Accessed on January 7, 2012.

9.  United States department of Agriculture. *Dietary Guidelines for Americans 2010. Foods and Food Components to Reduce*. 2010. Chapter 3. USDA;2010.

10. PCRM web site. Doctors Sue Federal Government for Deceptive Language on Meat, Dairy in New Dietary Guidelines. Available at: http://www.pcrm.org/media/news/doctors-sue-federal-government-for-deceptive. Accessed 1/7/2012. Accessed on January 15,2011.

11. Adams KM, Lindell KC, Kohlmeier M, Zeisel SH. Status of nutrition education in medical schools. *Am J Clin Nutr*. 2006;83(suppl)(4):941S-944S.

12. American Heart Association web site. 2011 Effectiveness-Based Guidelines for the Prevention of Cardiovascular Disease (CVD) in Women. Available at:

http://networking.americanheart.org/blogs/6/149 . Accessed on January 15,2011.

Chapter 6

1.  Park A. In 40 Years of Cancer Research, How Far Have We Come? *Time Healthland*(online). 2011;27. Available from http://healthland.time.com/2011/09/21/cancer-researchs-40th-anniversary-how-far-have-we-come/. Accessed on January 15,2011.

2.  Medscape web site. 40 Year War on Cancer. Can we win? Slide show. Available at: http://www.medscape.com/features/slideshow/war-on-cancer. Accessed on January 15,2011.

3.  American Cancer Society web site. Environmental Cancer Risks. Cancer Facts and Figures 2012. Available at: http://www.cancer.org/Research/CancerFactsFigures/CancerFactsFigures/cancer-facts-figures-2012. Accessed on January 22, 2012.

4.  Willett WC. Diet, nutrition, and avoidable cancer. *Environ Health Perspect.* 1995;66:1197-265.

5.  Butler TL, Fraser GE, Beeson WL, et al. Cohort Profile: The Adventist Health Study-2 (AHS-2). *Int j of Epidemiol.* 2008;37:260-265.

6.  T. Colin Campbell Foundation website. Cancer Facts-Meat Consumption and Cancer Risk. Available at: http://www.tcolincampbell.org/courses-resources/article/cancer-facts-meat-consumption-and-cancer-risk. Accessed on January 22, 2012.

7. Key TJ, Appleby PN, Spencer EA, et al. Cancer incidence in British vegetarians. *Br J Cancer*. 2009;101:192-197.

8. Thorogood M, Mann J, Appleby P, McPherson K. Risk of death from cancer and ischaemic heart disease in meat and non-meat eaters. *Br Med J*. 1994;308:1667-70.

9. Chang-Claude J, Frentzel-Beyme R, Eilber U. Mortality patterns of German vegetarians after 11 years of follow-up. *Epidemiology*. 1992;3:395-401.

10. Chang-Claude J, Frentzel-Beyme R. Dietary and lifestyle determinants among German vegetarians. *Int J Epidiom*. 1993;3:395-401.

11. Taylor EF, Burley VJ, Greenwood DC, Cade JE. Meat consumption and risk of breast cancer in the UK Women's Cohort Study. *Br J Cancer*. 2007;96:1139-1146.

12. Campbell TC. *The China Study*. Dallas, TX:BenBella Books, Inc; 2006.

13. Henning T, Kraus M, Brishwein M, Otto AM, Wolf B. Relevance of tumor microenvironment for progression, therapy, and drug development. *Anti-Cancer Drugs*. 2004;15:7-14

14. Brazier B. The Alkaline Advantage: How ph Promotes Optimal Health and Performance. *T.Colin Campbell Foundation website*. Available from:http://www.tcolincampbell.org/courses-resources/article/the-alkaline-advantage- how-ph-promotes-optimal-health-and-performance. Accessed on January 22, 2012.

15. Dictionary.com website. Available at: http://dictionary.reference.com/browse/mutagen. Accessed on January 25, 2012.

16. The Cancer Project Website. Cancer Facts-Meat Consumption and Cancer Risk. Available at: http://www.cancerproject.org/diet_cancer/facts/meat.php. Accessed on January 25, 2012.

17. Zheng W, Lee S. Well-Done Meat Intake, Heterocyclic Amine Exposure, and Cancer Risk. *Nutrition and Cancer.* 2009;61(4):437-446.

18. U.S. Department of Health and Human Services. Agency For Toxic Substances and Disease Registry Fact Sheet: Polycyclic Aromatic Hydrocarbons (PAHs). Available at: www.atsdr.cdc.gov/toxfaqs/tf.asp?id=121&tid=25 . Accessed on January 25, 2012.

19. Forman, D. Dietary exposure to N-nitroso compounds and the risk of human cancer. *Cancer Surv.* 1987;6(4):719-38.

20. American Cancer Society. ACS Guidelines on Nutrition and Physical Activity for Cancer Prevention. Available at: http://www.cancer.org/Healthy/EatHealthyGetActive/ACSGuidelinesonNutritionPhysicalActivityforCancerPrevention/acs-guidelines-on-nutrition-and-physical-activity-for-cancer-prevention-summary. Accessed on January 29, 2012.

21. American Institute of Cancer Research. http://www.aicr.org/reduce-your-cancer-risk/diet/

22. http://www.wcrf.org/cancer_facts/meat_consumption_patterns.php

## About the Author:

At a young age, Jennifer Moore observed her mother's presentation of a concern for healthy living. Running up and down the long halls of their old southern home, as treadmills were not the norm at that time, daily exercise proved to be essential for her mom. Following her mother's lead, as Jennifer grew, so did her love of health and wellness. Jennifer chose to study nutrition at Mississippi State University and went on to intern to become a Registered Dietitian at Vanderbilt University Medical Center in Nashville, TN. It was there that the idea of plant based nutrition was first introduced to her.

Professionally, Jennifer worked as a clinical dietitian in the specialty of nephrology. Personally, she tried to eat a plant based diet in the non-conducive environment of the deep-south. The more she worked and learned, the more convinced she became of the role that meat based diet practices play chronic disease development. After reviewing numerous studies while completing her Master's Degree through Central Michigan University, Jennifer fully embraced elimination of animal products in her diet. Her professors commented, "Jennifer, the research is overwhelmingly in your favor." She knew she had to teach the truths of this research; the truth that plant based nutrition preserves the health of humans more than any other diet regime. Animal based diets not only destroy health, but degrade God's creatures and destroy the environment. Join Jennifer on her health journey. Learn how you can impact the world one meal at a time.

# Visit www.Vegwell.com!

- Take affordable online classes to guide you with your plant based diet.

- Read Jenn's blog.

- Check out new recipes.

- Find out about upcoming events.

www.ingramcontent.com/pod-product-compliance
Lightning Source LLC
Chambersburg PA
CBHW070139290526
45789CB00002B/550